PYTHON FOR HEALTHCARE & MEDICAL RESEARCH

Hayden Van Der Post

Reactive Publishing

To my daughter, may she know anything is possible.

CONTENTS

Title Page

Dedication

Chapter 1. Introduction   1

Chapter 2. Python Basics   27

Chapter 3. Data Handling and Manipulation   56

Chapter 4. Data Visualization   80

Chapter 5. Data Preprocessing   108

Chapter 6. Statistical Analysis   130

Chapter 7. Machine Learning for Healthcare   156

Chapter 8. Deep Learning for Medical Imaging   181

Chapter 9. Natural Language Processing (NLP)   207

Chapter 10. Healthcare Data Ethics and Privacy   228

Chapter 11. Data Integration and Healthcare Systems   248

Chapter 12 Resources and Tools   273

Chapter 13. Conclusion   289

Appendix   296

Sample Code Snippets and Exercises   300

Additional Resources   304

CHAPTER 1.
INTRODUCTION

Unleashing the Power of Python in Healthcare and Medical Research

Imagine being able to analyze massive sets of healthcare data in a matter of seconds, predict disease outbreaks with remarkable accuracy, and revolutionize medical imaging with cutting-edge technology. What if I told you that all of this is possible, right now, with one of the world's most versatile and accessible programming languages: Python?

Welcome to "Python for Healthcare and Medical Research," a comprehensive journey into the exciting intersection of Python and the ever-evolving landscape of healthcare and medical science. In the following pages, we will embark on an exploration of how Python, a language renowned for its simplicity and power, is reshaping the healthcare industry and propelling medical research to new heights.

Are you a healthcare professional, a data analyst, a researcher, or simply someone with an insatiable curiosity about how technology is transforming the world of medicine? If so, this book is your gateway to a world where Python isn't just a programming language; it's a lifeline to better patient outcomes, faster drug discovery, and groundbreaking healthcare insights.

In this book, we will unveil the incredible capabilities of Python that allow you to analyze vast healthcare datasets with ease, create predictive models for disease detection, unlock the secrets hidden within medical images, and harness the potential of natural language processing in healthcare data. You will become proficient in the art of data handling, manipulation, visualization, and advanced analytics, and you'll discover the ethical considerations necessary to navigate the complex world of healthcare data.

Whether you're stepping into the realm of Python for the first time or you're an experienced coder seeking to deepen your expertise in healthcare and medical research, this book is your roadmap. Together, we'll dive into practical examples, case studies, and hands-on exercises that will empower you to drive innovation and positive change in the medical field using Python.

But this book isn't just about learning Python; it's about using it as a transformative tool to make a real impact on healthcare and medical research. Join us as we embark on this exciting journey, and let's unlock the limitless possibilities that Python offers in the realm of healthcare and medical discovery.

Why Python in Healthcare

In the realm of healthcare research, where innovation is not just a desire but a necessity, Python emerges as the unsung hero. Python, a versatile and powerful programming language, has been quietly revolutionizing the way we handle healthcare data, conduct medical research, and ultimately improve patient outcomes. As we delve into this chapter, let's explore the compelling reasons why Python has become the go-to choice for healthcare professionals and researchers worldwide.

Unveiling the Data Powerhouse:

Healthcare generates an avalanche of data daily, from electronic health records to medical imaging and patient histories. Python's ease of use and extensive libraries for data analysis make it the ideal tool for managing and making sense of this data deluge. Whether you're handling structured patient data or unstructured clinical notes, Python's robust libraries like Pandas and NumPy can transform raw data into meaningful insights with ease.

A Language for All Skill Levels:

One of Python's defining features is its accessibility. Seasoned data scientists and coding novices alike find Python welcoming. Its clean, readable syntax and extensive community support ensure that anyone, regardless of their background, can leverage Python to solve complex healthcare challenges. With Python, you don't need to be a coding wizard to perform data analytics and research; the language opens its doors to all.

Speed and Efficiency:

In the fast-paced world of healthcare, time is often the most critical factor. Python's efficiency shines through in data processing and analysis. Whether you're crunching numbers for a clinical trial or analyzing medical images in real-time, Python's speed, especially when optimized with libraries like

NumPy, offers a competitive advantage. It allows healthcare professionals to extract insights swiftly, making timely decisions for patient care.

Endless Libraries and Frameworks:

Python's library ecosystem is a treasure trove for healthcare professionals. The Scikit-Learn library empowers researchers to build intricate machine learning models for predicting disease outcomes, while libraries like Matplotlib and Seaborn facilitate data visualization, aiding in the clear presentation of results and patient data.

Interdisciplinary Collaboration:

In healthcare research, collaboration across various disciplines is vital. Python's adaptability enables it to be the common language for data scientists, clinicians, researchers, and engineers. The universality of Python breaks down communication barriers, ensuring that all stakeholders can participate in the analysis and interpretation of healthcare data.

Security and Reliability:

The healthcare sector places a premium on security and reliability. Python's extensive library support for secure coding practices and the ability to interface seamlessly with databases and data storage systems ensures the highest level of data integrity and patient privacy. It's a language that aligns perfectly with the stringent healthcare data regulations and standards.

Open Source and Cost-Effective:

In an era where cost-effectiveness is paramount, Python stands out as an open-source language that reduces overheads. It offers an extensive set of tools and libraries without the need for significant financial investments, making it an attractive choice for healthcare institutions aiming to optimize their research and data analysis processes.

Adaptability to Emerging Technologies:

Healthcare is continually evolving, and Python is keeping pace. It adapts seamlessly to emerging technologies like AI, deep learning, and natural language processing (NLP). As medical research continues to push boundaries, Python is there to support groundbreaking innovations in diagnostics, treatment, and patient care.

Python's presence in healthcare research is not just a trend; it's a fundamental shift in how we approach medical data, research, and patient well-being. In the following chapters, we will journey through the world of Python, exploring its capabilities and how it empowers healthcare professionals to drive advancements in medical science. Whether you're an experienced data scientist or a healthcare practitioner looking to harness the potential of Python, this book is your guide to mastering the language and using it to make a significant impact in the healthcare sector.

Let's embark on this transformative journey, where Python becomes not just a programming language but a vital tool for shaping the future of healthcare and medical research.

Book Structure and Goals

Now that we understand the compelling reasons why Python has become a key player in healthcare and medical research, let's take a moment to explore the organization of this book and its overarching objectives. By doing so, you'll gain a clear understanding of the roadmap we'll follow and the goals we aim to achieve throughout this journey.

A Guided Expedition:

This book, "Python for Healthcare and Medical Research," has been meticulously structured to provide you with a systematic and comprehensive learning experience. It's designed for readers of all levels, whether you're a healthcare professional, a data analyst, a researcher, or simply someone passionate about the intersection of technology and medicine.

Our primary goal is to empower you with the knowledge and skills required to leverage Python effectively in the healthcare domain. To achieve this, we've carefully organized the content into distinct chapters, each with a specific focus and set of objectives. Let's delve into the core structure of this book:

Chapter-by-Chapter Exploration:

The book is divided into sixteen chapters, each addressing a crucial aspect of Python's role in healthcare and medical research. These chapters are further divided into subsections, with each subsection serving as a building block for your understanding. Here's a glimpse of what you can expect in each chapter:Chapter 1: Introduction sets the stage, highlighting Python's significance in healthcare and medical research. We'll familiarize you with Python's role and its advantages in the field.

Chapter 2: Python Basics is your starting point, where we'll cover the fundamentals of Python. This chapter ensures that you have a solid foundation in the language before we dive deeper into healthcare-specific applications.

Chapters 3 to 9 delve into key healthcare topics. You'll explore data handling and manipulation, data visualization, data preprocessing, statistical analysis, machine learning, deep learning for medical imaging, and natural language processing (NLP). Each chapter equips you with the tools and knowledge required to tackle specific challenges within the healthcare domain.

Chapter 10: Healthcare Data Ethics and Privacy emphasizes the ethical considerations and privacy regulations surrounding healthcare data. Understanding these aspects is crucial for any professional working in the field.

Chapter 11: Data Integration and Healthcare Systems is dedicated to the integration of Python with electronic health record (EHR) systems and healthcare databases. It showcases the practical side of using Python in healthcare systems.

Chapter 12: Resources and Tools serves as a valuable reference, offering a compilation of healthcare datasets, Python libraries, online courses, and recommended conferences and communities.

Chapter 13: Conclusion summarizes the key takeaways from the book and encourages further exploration of Python in healthcare.

Chapter 14: Appendices includes a glossary of key terms, sample code snippets, and a list of references and citations for your reference.

Our Objectives:

Our primary objectives throughout this book are as follows:

Empower You: We aim to empower you with the knowledge and skills needed to excel in the healthcare and medical research domain using Python.

Bridge the Gap: We want to bridge the gap between the world of healthcare and the world of programming, ensuring that you have the necessary tools to make a significant impact in your field.

Provide Practical Guidance: We offer practical guidance, real-world examples, and hands-on exercises to reinforce your learning and understanding of Python's applications in healthcare.

Keep You Updated: With a focus on emerging technologies and trends, we ensure that you are well-prepared for the future of healthcare research.

As you progress through the chapters, you'll notice a steady accumulation of knowledge and skills, ultimately culminating in your ability to contribute to medical research, enhance patient care, and drive innovations using Python.

This book is more than just a guide; it's your companion in the fascinating world where Python meets healthcare. Together, we'll embark on a journey of exploration, discovery, and transformation. Whether you're an aspiring data scientist or a healthcare professional with a thirst for technological advancement, this book will equip you to thrive in the dynamic and ever-evolving field of healthcare and medical research.

Python's Role in Healthcare Research

In the vast landscape of healthcare and medical research, Python emerges as a powerful tool, catalyzing groundbreaking advancements and enabling intricate data analysis. This section serves as a gateway to understanding the pivotal role Python plays in the field, ranging from managing healthcare data to propelling medical breakthroughs.

Python has rapidly ascended to prominence in healthcare research for several compelling reasons. Let's delve into how this versatile programming language contributes to the ever-evolving world of medicine and data-driven healthcare.

Data Management and Analysis:

One of Python's standout attributes is its prowess in data management. In the healthcare sector, where data is abundant and multifaceted, Python shines brightly. Whether it's electronic health records (EHRs), patient data, clinical trial results, or medical images, Python serves as the bridge that connects these disparate data sources.

Python's extensive library ecosystem is instrumental in this regard. Libraries like Pandas and NumPy simplify data handling, offering efficient tools for data cleaning, preprocessing, and manipulation. These libraries ensure that healthcare professionals and researchers can work with data seamlessly, extracting valuable insights without the struggle of manual data wrangling.

Python also plays a crucial role in data visualization, which is paramount in healthcare research. Researchers can create informative and visually appealing plots and graphs to communicate their findings effectively. Libraries such as Matplotlib, Seaborn, and Plotly are indispensable when presenting data to medical professionals or the broader public.

Statistical Analysis and Machine Learning:

The realm of healthcare research thrives on statistical analysis. Python provides a rich ecosystem of statistical tools and packages. Researchers can perform descriptive statistics, analyze probability distributions, conduct hypothesis testing, examine correlations, and delve into advanced statistical methods with ease. Python's statistical libraries empower researchers to derive meaningful insights from healthcare data, ultimately contributing to more informed decision-making in clinical settings.

Machine learning is another area where Python excels. Healthcare professionals use Python to build predictive models, such as disease risk prediction and patient outcome forecasting. The Scikit-Learn library offers a wide array of algorithms for classification, regression, and clustering, tailored to the specific needs of healthcare applications. With machine learning, Python becomes a trusted ally in early disease detection, personalized medicine, and improving patient care.

Deep Learning for Medical Imaging:

The impact of Python in healthcare research is most profound in the domain of medical imaging. Deep learning, especially convolutional neural networks (CNNs), has revolutionized the interpretation of medical images like X-rays, MRIs, and CT scans. Python libraries such as TensorFlow and Keras facilitate the development of these cutting-edge deep learning models.

Deep learning models can accurately detect anomalies, identify tumors, and aid radiologists in providing more accurate diagnoses. Python's role in medical imaging is a testament to its transformative potential, illustrating how technology can enhance and streamline healthcare practices.

Natural Language Processing (NLP) for Healthcare:

Python extends its reach into the textual domain with natural language processing (NLP) applications. It's instrumental in analyzing clinical notes, research papers, and patient records. Python libraries like NLTK and spaCy enable the extraction of valuable information from unstructured text data.

Researchers leverage NLP to perform sentiment analysis, text classification, and named entity recognition within healthcare texts. Moreover, Python's capabilities extend to building healthcare chatbots and text analytics systems that automate processes and improve the efficiency of healthcare facilities.

In essence, Python's role in healthcare research is multifaceted. It supports the entire data lifecycle, from collection to analysis, and extends to making data-driven decisions, predicting patient outcomes, enhancing medical imaging, and processing clinical texts. Python empowers healthcare professionals and researchers to turn data into knowledge, ultimately advancing medical science and improving patient care. As we journey through the following chapters, you'll discover how to harness Python's capabilities for these critical healthcare applications.

Python is not just a programming language; it's a gateway to innovation in the ever-evolving world of healthcare and medical research. Whether you're a medical practitioner, a data scientist, or an enthusiast looking to make a meaningful impact, Python is your companion on this transformative journey. So, let's embark on this exploration of Python's capabilities in the context of healthcare, where each line of code has the potential to save lives and drive medical breakthroughs.

Setting Up Your Python Environment

Setting up your Python environment is the crucial first step on your journey to harnessing the power of Python in healthcare research. In this section, we'll provide you with a comprehensive guide on how to install and configure Python, ensuring you have the right tools at your disposal.

Installing Python

Python is known for its simplicity and versatility, making it an ideal choice for healthcare professionals and researchers. To get started, you'll first need to install Python on your system. Python is compatible with various operating systems, including Windows, macOS, and Linux. The following are the general steps to install Python:

Visit the Official Python Website: Open your web browser and go to the official Python website at www.python.org. Here, you can download the latest version of Python.

Choose the Right Version: Python has two major versions - Python 2 and Python 3. For this book, we recommend using Python 3, as it is the latest and most widely used version. Select the latest Python 3.x version available.

Downloading Python: Click on the download link for your chosen Python version and follow the on-screen instructions. The installer will guide you through the process, and you can choose to customize the installation if needed.

Adding Python to PATH: During installation, make sure to check the option to "Add Python to PATH." This is essential to run Python and its associated tools from the command line.

Verifying Installation: After the installation is complete, you can verify it by opening your command prompt or terminal and typing python --version. This should display the installed Python version.

Python Integrated Development Environments (IDEs)

Once Python is installed, you might want to use an Integrated Development Environment (IDE) to enhance your coding experience. An IDE provides a -friendly interface for writing and executing Python code. Some popular Python IDEs include:

PyCharm: Developed by JetBrains, PyCharm is a professional-grade Python IDE that offers features like code completion, debugging, and project management.

Visual Studio Code: VS Code is a lightweight yet powerful code editor that supports Python with the help of extensions.

It's highly customizable and widely used in the Python community.

Jupyter Notebook: If you're into data analysis and research, Jupyter Notebook is an excellent choice. It allows you to create and share documents that contain live code, equations, visualizations, and narrative text.

Configuring Your Environment

Configuring your Python environment involves setting up additional tools and libraries that are essential for healthcare research. This book will guide you through the installation of libraries like NumPy and Pandas, which are vital for data manipulation, and Matplotlib and Seaborn for data visualization. You'll also learn about virtual environments, a best practice for isolating your project dependencies.

In Python, you can create a virtual environment using the venv module. This isolates your project's dependencies, ensuring they don't interfere with other Python projects you might be working on. To create a virtual environment, you can follow these steps:

Open your command prompt or terminal.

Navigate to your project directory using the cd command.

Run python -m venv venv to create a virtual environment named "venv."

Once your virtual environment is created, you can activate it using the following commands:

On Windows: venv\Scripts\activate

On macOS and Linux: source venv/bin/activate

You'll notice that your command prompt or terminal prompt changes, indicating that the virtual environment is active.

In this section, you've learned how to install Python, select the right version, and configure your development environment. You're now equipped with the fundamental tools to dive into Python for healthcare and medical research.

Remember, a well-configured Python environment is the foundation for all the exciting Python applications we'll explore in this book. Whether you're analyzing healthcare data, building predictive models, or developing healthcare applications, a robust Python environment is your key to success.

Understanding the Healthcare Data Landscape

In the vast realm of healthcare, data is the lifeblood that fuels innovation, research, and decision-making. Understanding the diverse types of healthcare data and their significance is fundamental for anyone embarking on a journey to harness the power of Python in healthcare and medical research.

The Multifaceted World of Healthcare Data

Healthcare data comes in various forms, each serving a unique purpose and playing a vital role in improving patient care and medical research. To navigate this landscape effectively, it's crucial to grasp the nuances of the data types involved.

1. Electronic Health Records (EHR): EHRs are digital repositories of patient health information. They encompass everything from medical history and diagnoses to treatment plans and test results. Python's versatility is a perfect match for extracting, analyzing, and interpreting EHR data, enabling healthcare providers to make informed decisions and improving patient care.

2. Medical Imaging Data: Radiological images, such as X-rays, MRIs, and CT scans, are a goldmine of diagnostic information. Python, in conjunction with libraries like OpenCV and scikit-image, empowers researchers to process and analyze these images. For instance, convolutional neural networks (CNNs) can detect anomalies in medical images with remarkable accuracy, aiding in early disease diagnosis.

3. Clinical Trial Data: Clinical trials are the backbone of medical research, and they generate extensive datasets. Python's data manipulation capabilities, combined with libraries like Pandas and NumPy, facilitate the analysis of trial data. Researchers can identify trends, assess treatment efficacy, and ensure that new therapies meet rigorous standards.

4. Genomic Data: The Human Genome Project heralded an era of genomic data, where a single individual's DNA sequence can run into gigabytes of data. Python offers an array of tools and libraries for genomics research. With BioPython, scientists can analyze DNA sequences, study genetic variations, and gain insights into hereditary diseases.

5. Wearables and IoT Data: With the rise of wearables and the Internet of Things (IoT), healthcare data collection has extended beyond the clinical setting. Devices like smartwatches and fitness trackers continuously collect data

on heart rate, activity, and more. Python is instrumental in processing and making sense of this real-time data, enhancing remote patient monitoring and preventive healthcare.

Significance and Implications

The significance of comprehending this diverse healthcare data landscape cannot be overstated. It is the foundation upon which Python's capabilities are harnessed. Each data type mentioned above holds a key to better patient outcomes, more precise research, and improved decision-making.

Python's adaptability, combined with its extensive library support, makes it an indispensable tool for healthcare professionals and researchers. By leveraging Python, we can not only harness the power of this diverse data but also make it accessible, interpretable, and actionable.

As we delve deeper into the chapters of this book, you'll discover how Python can unlock the potential of each healthcare data type, offering you the skills and knowledge to embark on a transformative journey in the world of healthcare and medical research.

Remember, understanding the healthcare data landscape is just the beginning. The real magic happens when you dive into the practical implementation, and this book is your guide through that fascinating journey.

If you're eager to explore further, let's move on to Chapter 2, where we'll unravel the basics of Python and set the stage for our expedition into the realm of healthcare data analysis. But before we do that, let's understand why Python is becoming a ubiquitous presence in healthcare. So, without further ado, let's embark on our journey, where the Python programming language meets the intricate world of healthcare and medical research.

Health Data Challenges

In medical research, data plays an integral role in shaping the future of patient care, clinical advancements, and scientific breakthroughs. However, it's crucial to acknowledge that this treasure trove of health-related information comes with its unique set of challenges. In this section, we will delve into the intricacies of health data challenges, focusing on data quality and privacy – two aspects that are of paramount importance.

Data Quality: The Backbone of Healthcare Data

When it comes to healthcare, data quality isn't just a nice-to-have; it's absolutely essential. Inaccurate or incomplete data can lead to incorrect diagnoses, flawed research outcomes, and even jeopardize patient safety. To ensure data quality, healthcare professionals and data scientists must address several key challenges:

Data Accuracy: The accuracy of data is paramount. In healthcare, even the smallest error can have life-altering consequences. It's essential to implement robust data collection and validation processes to minimize inaccuracies.

Data Consistency: Healthcare data often originates from diverse sources such as electronic health records (EHRs), wearable devices, and laboratory results. Ensuring consistency across these sources is a significant challenge.

Data Completeness: Missing data can be a significant issue.

Patient records might have gaps, which can impact the continuity of care. Developing strategies for filling these gaps is critical.

Data Timeliness: In the fast-paced world of healthcare, timely access to data is crucial. Delays can hinder decision-making and research progress. Balancing speed with data integrity is a constant challenge.

To address these challenges, Python provides a versatile toolkit for data validation, cleaning, and transformation. Let's consider an example where we use Python to clean and validate patient data:

python

```python
import pandas as pd

# Load healthcare data
health_data = pd.read_csv('patient_records.csv')

# Checking for missing values
missing_values = health_data.isnull().sum()

# Handling missing values
# For instance, filling missing age values with the median age
of patients
median_age = health_data.median()
health_data.fillna(median_age, inplace=True)

# Check data accuracy - for example, ensuring blood pressure
readings are within reasonable limits
```

```
health_data = health_data >= 70) & (health_data <= 190)]
```

```
# Ensuring data consistency - standardizing gender labels
```

```
health_data.replace({'M': 'Male', 'F': 'Female', 'O': 'Other'},
inplace=True)
```

This Python code showcases how data quality challenges can be tackled within a healthcare dataset. By addressing missing values, ensuring accuracy, and maintaining consistency, we're taking significant steps to improve data quality.

Privacy Concerns in Healthcare Data

Healthcare data is not just sensitive; it's highly private. Patient information, medical records, and research data often contain sensitive details that must be protected. This subsection wouldn't be complete without addressing the privacy challenges in healthcare data management. Some of the key challenges include:

Patient Confidentiality: Healthcare providers and researchers must take extreme measures to protect patient confidentiality. Unauthorized access to patient data can lead to legal consequences and a loss of trust.

Compliance with Regulations: Regulations such as the Health Insurance Portability and Accountability Act (HIPAA) in the United States mandate strict rules on how healthcare data is collected, stored, and shared. Achieving compliance is a constant challenge.

Data Encryption: Ensuring data security through encryption and secure transmission methods is essential.

Encryption algorithms and protocols evolve, and staying up to date is a challenge.

Data Sharing: Collaboration among healthcare institutions and research organizations often necessitates sharing data. Finding the balance between sharing and safeguarding privacy is an ongoing challenge.

To demonstrate a Python approach to addressing privacy challenges, consider the following example:

```python
python

import pyAesCrypt
import os

# Encrypt a patient's medical record file
def encrypt_medical_record(file_path, password):
    # Define the output file
    encrypted_file = os.path.splitext(file_path) + '_encrypted' + os.path.splitext(file_path)

    # Encryption with AES-256
    bufferSize = 64 * 1024
    pyAesCrypt.encryptFile(file_path,          encrypted_file,
password, bufferSize)

    return encrypted_file

# Decrypt a patient's medical record file
def decrypt_medical_record(encrypted_file, password):
```

```python
    # Define the output file
    decrypted_file = os.path.splitext(encrypted_file) +
'_decrypted' + os.path.splitext(encrypted_file)

    # Decryption with AES-256
    bufferSize = 64 * 1024
    pyAesCrypt.decryptFile(encrypted_file, decrypted_file,
password, bufferSize)

    return decrypted_file
```

This Python code showcases how encryption can be used to protect sensitive healthcare data. The use of strong encryption methods is essential for safeguarding patient privacy.

The challenges related to healthcare data quality and privacy are complex and ever-evolving. Python, with its versatile libraries and frameworks, offers valuable tools to address these challenges effectively. By embracing the power of Python, healthcare professionals and data scientists can navigate the intricacies of healthcare data management while upholding data quality and patient privacy. As we progress through this book, we'll continue to explore the ways Python empowers us to overcome these challenges and drive innovations in healthcare and medical research.

As we conclude the introductory chapter of "Python for Healthcare & Medical Research," it's essential to reflect on the key insights we've gained so far. In this opening section, we embarked on a journey to explore the world of Python and its profound significance in healthcare and medical research. Let's take a moment to summarize the fundamental points that will set the stage for the exciting content that awaits you in the subsequent chapters.

Python, a versatile and -friendly programming language, has become a pivotal tool in the healthcare domain. Its popularity stems from its adaptability, which allows it to address a wide array of healthcare challenges. In our healthcare-driven world, it's imperative to recognize the increasing importance of Python, not only in data analysis but also in shaping the future of healthcare research.

With this book, our primary goal is to equip you with the knowledge and skills to harness the power of Python in healthcare. We aim to demystify the world of programming and ensure you are well-prepared to navigate the intricacies of healthcare data, analysis, and research. Whether you're a healthcare professional, a researcher, or a budding enthusiast, the content within these pages will empower you to leverage Python's capabilities effectively.

Our journey begins with understanding the structure of this book. We've meticulously organized the chapters to provide a logical progression of topics, ensuring that you build a solid foundation before delving into more complex subjects. The book is designed to cater to both beginners and experienced Python s, making it accessible to a broad audience.

We have set the stage for your learning experience, and in the chapters ahead, you'll find comprehensive insights into Python's role in healthcare research, data handling, manipulation, visualization, and statistical analysis. You will discover how Python can transform the way healthcare data is processed, interpreted, and analyzed. This journey isn't just about learning Python; it's about understanding how Python can revolutionize the healthcare industry.

In the following chapters, you'll dive into the basics of Python, learn about data types, variables, and control structures. You'll explore the essential elements of Python programming, including functions, modules, and error handling. As you progress, you'll gain an understanding of the significance of code readability and adherence to Python's style guide.

Subsequent sections will focus on data handling, manipulation, and visualization—crucial aspects of healthcare research. You'll master data cleaning techniques, learn how to work with healthcare data formats, and explore the world of data visualization using Python libraries like Matplotlib and Seaborn.

Data preprocessing is an indispensable skill, and our book provides in-depth knowledge of handling missing data, detecting outliers, scaling, and encoding categorical data. You'll become proficient in selecting the most relevant features from your medical datasets.

The journey doesn't stop there. We'll delve into the world of statistical analysis, where you'll uncover the importance of descriptive statistics, probability distributions, hypothesis testing, correlation analysis, and more in healthcare research.

Machine learning, a transformative force in healthcare, is the highlight of one of our chapters. You'll learn about Scikit-Learn, feature engineering, supervised and unsupervised learning techniques, model evaluation, and advanced topics in healthcare ML. These skills will empower you to build models that can predict diseases, assist in clinical decision-making, and more.

Deep learning, particularly in the context of medical imaging, is a game-changer. You'll explore convolutional neural networks (CNNs), image preprocessing, transfer learning, object detection, and segmentation, accompanied by practical case studies.

Natural Language Processing (NLP) has immense potential in healthcare, and our book will equip you with the skills to perform text preprocessing, sentiment analysis, text classification, named entity recognition, and even create healthcare chatbots.

The book goes beyond technical skills. You'll gain insights into healthcare data ethics and privacy, including privacy regulations, anonymization, and security strategies. You'll learn to navigate healthcare systems and integrate data from electronic health record systems, healthcare databases, and real-time data streams.

We've also prepared case studies that demonstrate Python's real-world applications in disease prediction, clinical trial analysis, medical image diagnosis, drug discovery, predictive analytics, and public health data analysis.

As we peer into the future, you'll be introduced to emerging technologies, the growing role of AI and ML in medical research, advancements in health informatics, and how Python contributes to shaping the future of healthcare research.

In closing, this chapter serves as the foundation upon which your Python journey in healthcare and medical research is built. Our mission is to empower you with the knowledge, tools, and skills needed to make a significant impact in the healthcare sector using Python. So, gear up for an exciting adventure as we embark on this transformative Python-driven healthcare odyssey. In the upcoming chapters, we'll delve into the heart of Python's applications in healthcare, ensuring you emerge as a proficient and confident Python practitioner in the medical field.

CHAPTER 2.
PYTHON BASICS

Python, often described as the Swiss Army knife of programming languages, serves as an indispensable tool in the world of healthcare and medical research. Its simplicity, versatility, and power have made it a primary choice for professionals in the field. In this section, we'll embark on a journey through the fundamental aspects of Python and discover why it has become a linchpin in healthcare applications.

Python: A Versatile Companion

Imagine a programming language that gracefully combines readability with functionality, and you're picturing Python. Its human-readable syntax makes it accessible, even for those new to coding. Python's motto, "Readability counts," exemplifies its dedication to straightforward, clean code.

This simplicity is a vital feature for healthcare professionals, where precision and clarity are paramount. When dealing with intricate medical data or conducting research, Python's syntax makes it easy to translate complex algorithms and procedures into code. This enhances communication, ensuring that all team members can understand and collaborate effectively.

Python's versatility knows no bounds. Whether you're diving into data analysis, machine learning, or working with healthcare databases, Python has libraries and tools to aid your endeavors. Libraries such as NumPy, Pandas, and Scikit-Learn empower you to manipulate data and build predictive models seamlessly. This versatility streamlines your workflow, allowing you to focus on the real challenges of healthcare and medical research.

The Power of an Open Source Community

Python's influence extends beyond its simplicity and versatility; it thrives due to its vibrant open-source community. Countless developers worldwide continually contribute to its growth. This extensive network of experts ensures that Python remains at the forefront of technology, with frequent updates, bug fixes, and the creation of new, innovative libraries.

In the realm of healthcare, this community is invaluable. Researchers and professionals can access an extensive library of open-source healthcare-related projects and tools. These resources facilitate everything from advanced imaging analysis to natural language processing for electronic health records (EHR).

Python's Role in Healthcare

Python is not only about coding; it's about driving innovation in healthcare and medical research. Its applications span a wide spectrum of vital functions:

Data Analysis: Python's libraries for data analysis, such

as Pandas and NumPy, help healthcare professionals extract valuable insights from massive datasets. This is crucial for making informed decisions and drawing meaningful conclusions from complex medical data.

Machine Learning: Python's Scikit-Learn library enables the creation of predictive models, disease detection algorithms, and patient outcome analysis. Machine learning algorithms can identify patterns and trends in healthcare data, contributing to early diagnosis and improved patient care.

Medical Imaging: In the field of medical imaging, Python's libraries like OpenCV and PyDicom allow professionals to process, analyze, and visualize medical images with ease. This is pivotal for tasks such as tumor detection, organ segmentation, and tracking disease progression.

Natural Language Processing (NLP): For electronic health records and clinical notes, Python's NLP libraries like NLTK and spaCy can perform sentiment analysis, information extraction, and named entity recognition. This is indispensable for automating data extraction and analysis in healthcare documents.

Healthcare System Integration: Python's ability to develop APIs and interfaces facilitates integration with electronic health record (EHR) systems, databases, and real-time data streams. This seamless connectivity enhances the efficiency of healthcare processes and supports better patient care.

Python: A Vital Skill

In healthcare and medical research, proficiency in Python is not just an asset; it's a competitive advantage. Whether you're a medical professional aiming to automate data analysis, a researcher exploring the potential of machine learning, or a developer creating innovative healthcare solutions, Python is the bridge that connects your vision to reality.

As we delve deeper into this book, you will discover the tools and techniques that empower you to harness the full potential of Python in healthcare. With its simplicity, versatility, and a community of like-minded professionals and researchers, Python is your companion on the journey to improved healthcare and medical discoveries.

Now that you've got a glimpse of Python's power and versatility, it's time to delve into the specifics. In the subsequent chapters, we will explore Python's core components, essential data handling techniques, and its role in transforming healthcare. Stay with us on this remarkable journey as we unlock the secrets of Python for healthcare and medical research. The world of possibilities awaits you, and Python will be your guiding light.

Let's get started with the basics of Python and build a strong foundation for our journey ahead.

Variables and Data Types

In the world of Python, understanding variables and data types is akin to mastering the alphabet before diving into writing eloquent prose. Just as an author crafts their story with carefully chosen words, a Python programmer weaves their code with the right data types and variables. In this section, we'll unravel the art of Python data types and variable usage.

Python, being a dynamically-typed language, allows you to work with various data types without declaring them explicitly. Let's explore the fundamental data types that underpin Python's versatility.

Integers (int): These are your whole numbers, both positive and negative. They are the building blocks for numerical operations in Python. For instance, if you're dealing with a patient's age, you'd use an integer data type.

python

patient_age = 35

Floating-Point Numbers (float): When precision is required, floating-point numbers come into play. They represent real numbers and are indispensable for anything from calculating drug dosages to analyzing sensor data.

python

body_temperature = 98.6

Strings (str): Textual data is ubiquitous in healthcare, from patient names to clinical notes. Strings in Python are your go-to data type for handling such information.

python

patient_name = "John Doe"

Booleans (bool): Healthcare often involves making binary

decisions, like whether a test result is positive or negative. Booleans are perfect for such scenarios, representing either True or False.

python

test_result = True

Now, let's dive into variable usage. In Python, a variable is a symbolic name associated with a value. These variables serve as placeholders, storing data that can be manipulated, analyzed, and processed.

For instance, imagine you're conducting a clinical study, and you want to keep track of patient blood pressure readings. You can create variables to store this information:

python

patient_1_bp = 120/80
patient_2_bp = 135/90

In the example above, patient_1_bp and patient_2_bp are variables that hold the blood pressure values for two patients. These variables allow you to perform various operations, such as calculating averages or identifying trends.

Python's flexibility shines when variables are combined with data types. You can store any data type in a variable, and Python will adjust accordingly. Here's an example:

python

```
patient_id = 12345
patient_name = "Alice"
patient_age = 42
```

In the code above, patient_id holds an integer, patient_name stores a string, and patient_age is an integer. Python doesn't require explicit data type declarations, making it convenient for developers.

Let's delve deeper and explore data type conversion. Python allows you to change the data type of a variable when needed. For example, you might want to convert a patient's age from an integer to a string for display purposes:

python

```
patient_age = 28
patient_age_str = str(patient_age)
```

In this snippet, str(patient_age) converts the integer 28 into the string "28". It's a handy feature for formatting data as required.

To sum up, understanding Python's data types and variable usage is fundamental in your journey to harness the power of Python in healthcare and medical research. Just as a writer needs to select the right words and arrange them coherently, a Python programmer must choose the appropriate data types and employ variables effectively to process healthcare data seamlessly. This knowledge forms the foundation upon which you'll build your expertise as we progress through this book.

Loops: Unleashing the Power of Repetition

Loops are the workhorses of programming, allowing you to perform a set of actions multiple times without having to write the same code over and over. Python provides two main types of loops: the for loop and the while loop.

The for loop is ideal when you want to iterate over a sequence, such as a list, tuple, or string. It allows you to execute a block of code for each item in the sequence. Here's an example of a simple for loop:

python

```
fruits =
for fruit in fruits:
    print(fruit)
```

In this code, we create a list of fruits and use a for loop to iterate through each item in the list and print it to the screen.

On the other hand, the while loop is used when you want to repeat a block of code as long as a certain condition is met. Here's a basic example:

python

```
count = 0
while count < 5:
    print("Count is", count)
    count += 1
```

In this code, the while loop continues to execute as long as the count variable is less than 5. It increments the count in each iteration.

Conditionals: Making Decisions

Conditionals in Python are your tools for making decisions within your code. They help your program take different paths based on whether a condition is true or false. The primary conditional statements in Python are if, elif (short for "else if"), and else.

Here's a straightforward example of an if statement:

python

```
age = 18
if age >= 18:
    print("You are an adult.")
```

In this code, we check if the variable age is greater than or equal to 18. If it is, we print "You are an adult."

The elif statement allows you to check multiple conditions in sequence:

python

```
temperature = 25
if temperature > 30:
    print("It's hot outside.")
```

```python
elif temperature > 20:
    print("It's a pleasant day.")
else:
    print("It's a bit chilly.")
```

In this example, we evaluate the temperature and print a message based on different temperature ranges.

The else statement provides a default action to take when none of the previous conditions are met. It serves as the "catch-all" option.

These are just the tip of the iceberg when it comes to control structures in Python. Loops and conditionals are powerful tools that allow you to create flexible, responsive, and efficient code. In this chapter, we'll explore more complex examples and practical use cases to help you master these essential programming concepts.

For those of you eager to dive into coding, let's put these concepts into action with some hands-on Python examples.

Python Code Example:

Let's use a for loop to calculate the sum of all numbers from 1 to 10:

python

```python
total = 0
for num in range(1, 11):
    total += num
```

print("The sum of numbers from 1 to 10 is:", total)

With these fundamental control structures at your disposal, you're well on your way to becoming proficient in Python programming. The ability to loop through data and make decisions based on conditions is crucial for handling real-world problems in healthcare and medical research. In the subsequent chapters, we'll apply these concepts to real healthcare data, unlocking the full potential of Python in this domain.

The Power of Functions

Picture a healthcare facility where doctors, nurses, and various specialists work together seamlessly to provide care. Each individual possesses a specific set of skills and responsibilities. Functions in Python can be likened to these specialists in the healthcare ecosystem. They are self-contained units of code designed to perform specific tasks, and they play a vital role in keeping your code organized and manageable.

Here's a simple Python function to compute the BMI (Body Mass Index) of a patient based on their weight and height:

python

```python
def calculate_bmi(weight, height):
    """Calculate BMI (Body Mass Index)."""
    bmi = weight / (height ** 2)
    return bmi
```

In this example, calculate_bmi is a function that takes two

parameters, weight and height, and returns the computed BMI. Functions are encapsulated, meaning they can be easily reused throughout your code, just as healthcare professionals utilize their specialized skills in various patient scenarios.

The Modular Approach

Now, let's shift our focus to modules. Modules in Python are collections of related functions, variables, and classes. In healthcare, think of modules as specialized departments within a hospital, such as cardiology or radiology. Each module has its own unique functions and components but operates within the broader healthcare system.

Python's standard library provides a rich set of modules that are indispensable for healthcare applications. For instance, the math module offers functions for mathematical operations, which can be invaluable when dealing with medical data.

Here's a snippet that shows how to use functions from the math module:

python

```python
import math

# Calculate the square root of a patient's age
age = 49
sqrt_age = math.sqrt(age)
```

In this example, we import the math module and use its sqrt function to compute the square root of a patient's age. By organizing related functions into modules, your code becomes more structured and easier to maintain, just as healthcare departments streamline their operations.

The Significance of Modular Code

In the healthcare field, patient records are well-structured to ensure quick access to critical information. Similarly, in Python programming, maintaining modular code is crucial for the efficient development, debugging, and scalability of healthcare applications.

Modular code allows you to compartmentalize different aspects of your healthcare project. You might have a module for data analysis, one for data visualization, and another for machine learning models. This division of labor mirrors how healthcare institutions have specialized departments for various medical disciplines.

Furthermore, when you need to update or troubleshoot a specific aspect of your code, you can focus your attention on the relevant module without affecting other parts of your application. This compartmentalization makes your code more robust and sustainable, a trait highly desirable in healthcare, where precision and reliability are paramount.

In summary, functions and modules are the healthcare heroes of Python programming. Functions perform specific tasks like skilled healthcare professionals, and modules organize related functions into specialized units, just as healthcare departments streamline patient care. Embracing this modular approach allows you to create robust, maintainable, and efficient Python code that's essential for healthcare and medical research applications.

With these concepts in mind, you're now equipped to explore the fascinating world of Python for healthcare with a solid foundation in functions and modules. In the subsequent chapters, you'll delve deeper into the practical applications of Python in healthcare and medical research, building upon the principles introduced here.

Reading from Files

To begin, let's consider a common scenario: you have a dataset in a file, and you want to analyze its contents. Python provides various ways to read from files, making it a versatile tool for data extraction. Let's start with one of the most straightforward methods using Python's built-in functions.

python

```
# Opening a file in read mode
with open('data.txt', 'r') as file:
    contents = file.read()
    print(contents)
```

In the example above, we use the open function with the file name and the mode 'r', which stands for read. The with statement ensures the file is properly closed after use. We read the file's content and print it to the console.

Additionally, Python allows reading files line by line:

python

```
# Reading a file line by line
with open('data.txt', 'r') as file:
    for line in file:
        print(line)
```

This method is especially useful for large files as it consumes minimal memory.

Writing to Files

Now, consider the scenario in which you want to store your results or insights in a file. Python makes this process straightforward as well. Here's how you can write to a file:

python

```
# Opening a file in write mode
with open('results.txt', 'w') as file:
    file.write("These are the results of our analysis.")
```

In the code above, we open the file in write mode using 'w'. Be cautious when using write mode, as it will overwrite the file's content if it already exists. If you want to add content to an existing file, you can use 'a' mode for append.

Handling File Paths

When working with files, you'll often need to deal with different file locations. It's essential to understand how to handle file paths in a way that's platform-independent. Python's os module can help you with this.

python

```python
import os

# Joining file paths
folder = 'data'
filename = 'file.txt'
file_path = os.path.join(folder, filename)

# Opening a file using the path
with open(file_path, 'r') as file:
    content = file.read()
```

In this example, we use os.path.join() to create a platform-independent path to our file, which is particularly useful when your code needs to run on different operating systems.

Error Handling with Files

In real-world applications, it's crucial to anticipate potential errors when working with files. For instance, a file you intend to read might not exist, or you might not have the necessary permissions. Python allows you to handle such situations gracefully with try and except blocks.

python

```python
try:
    with open('nonexistent.txt', 'r') as file:
        content = file.read()
```

except FileNotFoundError:

   print("The file does not exist.")

This is a simplified example, but it showcases how to handle specific exceptions, in this case, a FileNotFoundError.

Remember, as you work with real healthcare data, you may need more advanced error handling to ensure the security and integrity of the data you're dealing with.

Exception Handling

In the world of programming, we often encounter situations where things don't go as planned. This is where exception handling comes into play, as it allows us to anticipate and gracefully deal with unexpected errors in our Python code.

Understanding Exceptions:

Before we delve into the practical aspects of exception handling, let's first understand what exceptions are. In Python, an exception is an event that occurs during the execution of a program that disrupts the normal flow of instructions. These exceptions can be triggered by various factors, such as invalid input, file not found, or even attempting operations like division by zero.

Imagine you are writing code to read data from a file, and that file doesn't exist. Without proper exception handling, your program would simply crash, leaving you with an error message. Exception handling enables you to intercept these errors and take specific actions to address them, making your code more robust and -friendly.

Using Try and Except:

The cornerstone of exception handling in Python is the "try" and "except" block. Here's how it works:

python

```
try:
    # Code that might raise an exception
    result = 10 / 0
except ZeroDivisionError:
    # Code to handle the exception
    print("You can't divide by zero!")
```

In this example, the code inside the "try" block attempts to divide 10 by 0, which is a clear error. However, instead of crashing, the program gracefully proceeds to the "except" block and prints a -friendly error message.

Types of Exceptions:

Python provides a wide range of built-in exceptions, each designed for specific types of errors. These include:

ZeroDivisionError: Raised when attempting to divide by zero.

FileNotFoundError: Raised when a specified file does not exist.

TypeError: Raised when an operation is performed on an

object of inappropriate type.

ValueError: Raised when a function receives an argument of the correct type but an inappropriate value.

NameError: Raised when trying to access a local or global variable that hasn't been defined.

And many more.

Custom Exceptions:

While Python offers an extensive list of predefined exceptions, you can also create your own custom exceptions by subclassing the built-in "Exception" class. This allows you to handle application-specific errors elegantly. For instance:

python

```python
class MyCustomError(Exception):
    def __init__(self, message):
        super().__init__(message)

try:
    # Code that might raise a custom exception
    raise MyCustomError("This is a custom exception!")
except MyCustomError as e:
    print(f"Caught an exception: {e}")
```

Final Thoughts:

Exception handling is a critical aspect of writing robust and reliable Python code, especially in healthcare and medical research applications, where data accuracy and integrity are paramount. By proactively addressing potential issues, you ensure that your program continues running smoothly even in the face of unexpected challenges.

In practice, a good approach is to handle different exceptions separately, providing informative error messages and taking appropriate actions. By doing so, you not only make your code more -friendly but also aid in the debugging process.

Exception handling is a fundamental skill for any Python developer. It enables you to foresee and address potential pitfalls, making your code resilient in the face of unforeseen circumstances. As we progress through this book, you'll find numerous real-world examples of exception handling tailored to the specific challenges encountered in healthcare and medical research. So, stay tuned and let's explore the fascinating world of Python in healthcare.

Python Best Practices

Welcome to Python Best Practices, a segment where we delve into the art of writing Python code that not only works but also shines with clarity and maintainability. In the world of programming, crafting efficient and elegant code is akin to creating a work of art. Just like a skilled painter employs different brush strokes and shades to create a masterpiece, a proficient programmer uses best practices to sculpt a codebase that's easy to understand and extend.

Consistency is Key

Let's start with a fundamental principle: consistency. Consistency in your code is like the backbone of a sturdy building. It provides structure and ensures that your code is predictable. This means adhering to the PEP 8 style guide, Python's style bible. PEP 8 outlines conventions for formatting your code, from indentation to variable naming. Ensuring that your code conforms to these conventions makes it easier for you and other developers to read and maintain.

python

```python
# Inconsistent
def calculate_total(items):
Total = 0
for item in items:
total += item
```

```python
# Consistent (PEP 8)
def calculate_total(items):
    total = 0
    for item in items:
        total += item
```

Modular Design

Divide and conquer, a strategy used throughout history, also applies to coding. Your code should be modular, meaning it's broken down into small, manageable components. Each module should have a single responsibility, making it easier to test and maintain.

python

```python
# Not Modular
```

```python
def process_data(data):
    # A long and complex function
```

```python
# Modular
def validate_data(data):
    # Ensure data is in the correct format
```

```python
def clean_data(data):
    # Clean and transform data
```

```python
def analyze_data(data):
    # Perform data analysis
```

```python
def visualize_data(data):
    # Generate visualizations
```

Documentation and Comments

Imagine you're a tour guide leading a group through a dense forest. Documentation is your map and comments are the signposts. They guide you and others through your codebase. Every function, class, and complex piece of code should be well-documented. Docstrings are an excellent way to explain the purpose and usage of functions and classes.

python

```python
def calculate_total(items):
    """
    Calculate the total sum of a list of items.
```

Args:

   items (list): A list of numeric items.

Returns:

   float: The total sum of the items.

"""

total = 0

for item in items:

   total += item

return total

Testing and Test-Driven Development (TDD)

Testing is like quality control for your code. By writing tests, you ensure that your code works as expected and that future changes don't break existing functionality. Test-Driven Development (TDD) is a practice where you write tests before writing the actual code. It may seem counterintuitive, but it forces you to think about the expected behavior and interface of your code first.

```python
import unittest

def add(a, b):
    return a + b

class TestAddition(unittest.TestCase):
    def test_addition(self):
```

```
    self.assertEqual(add(2, 3), 5)
```

Version Control with Git

In the world of coding, mistakes are inevitable. That's where version control comes into play. Git is a version control system that allows you to track changes to your code, collaborate with others, and recover from errors. It's an indispensable tool for any serious developer.

Optimizing Code

Efficiency is crucial, especially when working with large datasets or resource-intensive operations. Profiling tools like cProfile can help you identify bottlenecks in your code. This data-driven approach ensures you focus your optimization efforts where they matter most.

python

```python
import cProfile

def slow_function():
    result = 0
    for i in range(10**6):
        result += i
    return result

cProfile.run('slow_function()')
```

Significance of Code Readability

In the world of healthcare and medical research, the importance of code readability cannot be overstated. Python has emerged as a go-to language in this domain, and there are compelling reasons behind this choice. The simplicity and readability of Python's syntax make it an ideal candidate for professionals who may not have extensive programming backgrounds.

Consider this: Python's clean and straightforward syntax enables healthcare researchers, doctors, and data scientists to focus more on solving complex medical problems and less on deciphering convoluted code. When dealing with issues of life and health, the last thing you want is to be puzzled by your own or your colleague's code.

Readable code facilitates collaboration and understanding, allowing multiple professionals to work on projects with ease. In healthcare research, collaboration is often the norm, and readability becomes a lifeline in this context. Whether it's building predictive models, analyzing patient data, or developing healthcare systems, Python's readability fosters teamwork.

Adherence to PEP 8:

Python Enhancement Proposal 8, or PEP 8 for short, is the style guide for Python code. It's a set of conventions and guidelines for writing clean, readable, and maintainable Python code. Think of it as a recipe book for coding in Python, ensuring consistency across your projects and with the broader Python community.

PEP 8 covers a wide array of topics, from indentation

and whitespace to naming conventions and even how to handle imports. By following PEP 8, you make your code comprehensible not just to you but to every Python developer who may encounter your work. It's like speaking a common language, and in the context of healthcare research, where precision and clarity are paramount, this common language is invaluable.

Let's take a moment to look at a brief example that underscores the significance of code readability and PEP 8 adherence. Consider two code snippets that aim to achieve the same task:

Non-Compliant Code:

python

```
def get_patientDetails(patientId):
    try:
    file = open("patient_data.txt","r")
        data = file.read()
        details = data.split(";")
    return details
    except:
        print('Error reading data!')
    return None
```

PEP 8 Compliant Code:

python

```
def get_patient_details(patient_id):
```

```python
try:
    with open("patient_data.txt", "r") as file:
        data = file.read()
        details = data.split(";")
        return details
except FileNotFoundError as e:
    print(f'Error reading data: {e}')
    return None
```

In the compliant code, you can immediately see the difference. It's neatly organized, follows naming conventions (snake_case for functions and variables), uses consistent indentation, and handles exceptions gracefully. This adherence to PEP 8 not only makes the code easier to read but also enhances its reliability and maintainability.

Understanding the Power of Python: Python is a versatile and - friendly programming language. We've seen how its simplicity and readability make it an ideal choice for beginners. Its extensive standard library and vast community support offer numerous resources to learners and practitioners alike.

Variables and Data Types: We delved into the fundamentals of Python's data types and variables. Understanding these concepts is crucial as they form the building blocks of any Python program. Variables are like containers that store data, and different data types determine the kind of information we can store.

Control Structures: We explored control structures, including loops and conditionals. These constructs are essential for controlling the flow of your Python programs. Loops allow us to execute a set of statements repeatedly, while conditionals enable us to make decisions within our code.

Functions and Modules: We introduced the concept of functions, which are reusable blocks of code. Python's modular approach allows us to break our code into smaller, manageable pieces, making it easier to read, maintain, and collaborate with others.

Working with Files: Python is incredibly powerful when it comes to handling files. We discussed how to read from and write to files, a skill you'll often need in real-world applications.

Exception Handling: Dealing with errors and exceptions is a vital part of programming. We learned how Python enables us to gracefully handle errors through exception handling, making our programs more robust.

Best Practices and PEP 8: Adhering to best practices and Python's style guide, PEP 8, is crucial for writing clean and maintainable code. We emphasized the importance of good coding habits and following conventions to make your code more readable and collaborative.

In summary, the Python basics chapter has laid a strong foundation for your journey into Python programming. You've grasped the core concepts, and now it's time to put them into practice in your healthcare and medical research projects. Remember that learning a new language, especially one as versatile as Python, is a journey that requires practice and dedication.

As you move forward in your Python for Healthcare

and Medical Research adventure, keep these fundamental principles in mind. Python is a powerful tool that will open doors to endless possibilities in the field of healthcare. Whether you're analyzing medical data, building predictive models, or working with healthcare systems, your understanding of Python basics will serve as a solid platform for your future endeavors.

So, embrace your newfound knowledge, explore, and don't hesitate to experiment with the code examples provided. The best way to learn is by doing. The Python basics chapter is just the beginning of your exciting journey into the world of healthcare and medical research powered by Python. Stay curious, stay determined, and keep coding!

CHAPTER 3. DATA HANDLING AND MANIPULATION

In healthcare and medical research, the data generated is nothing short of colossal. From electronic health records to medical imaging, healthcare data encompasses a vast landscape. But what does one do with this sea of information? That's where data handling steps onto the stage, the unsung hero that takes this raw data and transforms it into actionable insights.

The Vital Role of Data Handling

Before we dive into the intricate world of data handling, it's crucial to understand why it's so pivotal in the context of healthcare and medical research. Imagine you have a treasure chest filled with precious gems, but it's locked tight. Data handling is the key that unlocks this chest, revealing the valuable insights hidden within.

The importance of data handling in healthcare can't be overstated. It's the process of collecting, cleaning, organizing, and transforming data into a format that's suitable for analysis. This preparatory phase ensures that the data you're working with is accurate, consistent, and relevant. Healthcare decisions, diagnosis, and research outcomes all depend on the quality of the data used, making data handling the cornerstone of success.

Let's illustrate this with a simple example. Imagine a hospital collects patient data for research purposes. This data includes various attributes like age, gender, medical history, and test results. Data handling involves tasks such as verifying that the data is complete (no missing values), correcting errors, and structuring it in a way that's easy to analyze. These processes are like cleaning the gems in our treasure chest, ensuring they shine brightly.

Data Handling in Action

Python, the star of our book, offers an arsenal of tools and libraries that make data handling an efficient and streamlined process. With Python, you can perform tasks such as data cleansing, transformation, and even integration with different data sources. The power of Python lies in its simplicity and versatility, enabling even those new to programming to become adept at handling complex healthcare data.

Let's take a practical look at Python in action with a sample code snippet. This example demonstrates how to load a CSV file containing healthcare data, examine its structure, and clean it by handling missing values:

python

import pandas as pd

Load the healthcare data from a CSV file

```
data = pd.read_csv('healthcare_data.csv')

# Check for missing values
missing_values = data.isnull().sum()

# Fill missing values with appropriate methods
data.fillna(data.median(), inplace=True)
data.fillna('Not available', inplace=True)

# Data is now clean and ready for analysis
```

In this code, we import the Pandas library, which is a powerhouse for data handling in Python. We load the healthcare data from a CSV file and use Pandas to check for missing values and fill them with suitable replacements.

The Road Ahead

As we journey through this book, you'll gain a deeper understanding of data handling, including techniques for data cleaning, preprocessing, and integration. You'll become proficient in using Python libraries like Pandas and NumPy to manipulate healthcare data efficiently.

Remember, data handling is the first step in unlocking the potential of healthcare data. In the chapters that follow, we'll explore more advanced data handling techniques and delve into the world of data manipulation, but it all starts here, with the fundamentals.

NumPy's Role in Healthcare Data

NumPy excels in numerical and array-based operations. Its ability to handle large, multi-dimensional arrays and matrices is particularly relevant in the healthcare domain, where data often comes in complex formats. Whether you're dealing with medical images, patient records, or clinical trial data, NumPy simplifies the process of data manipulation.

One of NumPy's primary advantages is its speed. Behind the scenes, NumPy operations are executed in highly optimized C code, making it significantly faster than standard Python lists. When processing large datasets or performing complex mathematical computations, this speed is crucial.

Getting Started with NumPy

Before we dive into the world of healthcare data manipulation using NumPy, it's essential to understand the basics. NumPy can be easily integrated into your Python environment through installation using tools like pip or conda. Once installed, you can import it into your Python script or Jupyter Notebook with the following line of code:

python

import numpy as np

The alias np is a common convention used among data scientists and programmers. It simplifies the process of calling NumPy functions and methods.

Creating NumPy Arrays

At the core of NumPy is the numpy.ndarray, an efficient data structure for handling arrays. You can create NumPy arrays from Python lists or other iterable objects. For example, to create a simple array, you can use the following code:

python

import numpy as np

my_list =
my_array = np.array(my_list)

Now, 'my_array' is a NumPy array.

NumPy arrays can have multiple dimensions, making them suitable for various healthcare data types, such as time-series data, 2D medical images, or even 3D scans. Creating multi-dimensional arrays is straightforward:

python

import numpy as np

two_d_array = np.array(,])

Basic Operations with NumPy

NumPy offers a wide range of functions and methods for array manipulation. Here are some common operations you'll encounter in healthcare data analysis:

Element-wise Operations: NumPy simplifies element-wise operations, making it easy to perform calculations on entire arrays without explicit loops. For example, you can add two arrays element-wise as follows:

python

```
import numpy as np

array1 = np.array()
array2 = np.array()

result = array1 + array2
```

Aggregations: NumPy provides functions for calculating statistics on arrays, such as mean, median, standard deviation, and more. For instance:

python

```
import numpy as np

data = np.array()

mean = np.mean(data)
median = np.median(data)
```

Array Slicing: Slicing NumPy arrays allows you to extract specific elements or subarrays. This is particularly useful for selecting relevant portions of healthcare data:

python

import numpy as np

data = np.array()

# Extract the elements from index 2 to 4 (exclusive).
subset = data

These are just the tip of the iceberg when it comes to NumPy's capabilities. It offers a wide array of mathematical, logical, and statistical functions to suit your healthcare data needs.

Pandas

In the vast landscape of healthcare data, efficient handling and manipulation of data are paramount. This is where the Pandas library steps in as a game-changer. Pandas, a powerful data manipulation and analysis library for Python, equips you with the tools you need to work with complex healthcare datasets.

Why Pandas?

Imagine having to navigate and make sense of extensive medical records, clinical data, and research findings. Pandas simplifies this intricate process, allowing you to explore, clean, and analyze data with ease. But before we delve into the practical aspects, let's take a moment to understand why Pandas is indispensable in healthcare research.

Healthcare data is often unstructured, messy, and diverse,

comprising patient information, laboratory results, diagnostic reports, and more. Pandas, with its data structures, Series and DataFrames, provides a unified way to organize this diverse data. It's like having a versatile toolbox that can adapt to any data format you throw at it.

Getting Acquainted with Pandas

To embark on your journey with Pandas, you first need to import the library into your Python environment. If you've been following along from Chapter 1, you should already have Python set up. Now, let's explore a basic Pandas introduction:

python

import pandas as pd

In the above code, we imported Pandas as 'pd,' which is a common convention among Pandas s. This allows us to access Pandas functions and methods using 'pd' as a prefix.

Creating DataFrames

In healthcare research, you'll typically work with structured data. The primary data structure in Pandas is the DataFrame. It resembles a table with rows and columns. You can create a DataFrame from various sources, such as CSV files, databases, or by directly inputting data.

python

# Creating a simple DataFrame
data = {'Patient_ID': ,

```
    'Age': ,
    'Diagnosis': }
```

df = pd.DataFrame(data)

With this DataFrame, you can now perform a multitude of operations like filtering patients based on their age, grouping by diagnosis, or even conducting statistical analyses.

Data Cleaning and Transformation

Healthcare data is notorious for containing missing values or inconsistencies. Pandas simplifies the process of data cleaning and transformation. Here's an example of how you can handle missing data:

python

```
# Handling missing data
df.fillna(df.mean(), inplace=True)
```

In the above code, we fill missing age values with the mean age of patients. This ensures that our dataset remains complete and reliable for further analysis.

Exploratory Data Analysis

One of the first steps in healthcare research is to gain insights from your data. Pandas provides a multitude of functions to help you with exploratory data analysis. For instance, you can quickly get an overview of your dataset's statistics:

python

```
# Summary statistics
summary = df.describe()
```

This code generates statistics like count, mean, standard deviation, and more for numerical columns, giving you a snapshot of your data.

Data Visualization

While data manipulation is the heart of healthcare research, data visualization is its soul. Pandas can seamlessly integrate with data visualization libraries like Matplotlib and Seaborn to help you create insightful graphs and plots. Here's a simple example of how you can visualize age distribution:

python

```
import matplotlib.pyplot as plt

# Creating a histogram
df.plot(kind='hist', bins=10, title='Age Distribution')
plt.xlabel('Age')
plt.ylabel('Frequency')
plt.show()
```

This code generates a histogram showing the distribution of ages in your dataset.

Practical Implementation

Now that we've covered the fundamentals, it's time to get hands-on experience. In this chapter, we'll walk you through practical exercises, where you'll apply Pandas to real healthcare data scenarios. Whether it's analyzing patient records, tracking disease trends, or studying treatment outcomes, Pandas will be your trusted companion.

Remember, Pandas isn't just a tool; it's your key to unlocking the insights hidden within healthcare data. With Pandas, you have the power to manipulate, analyze, and visualize your way to groundbreaking discoveries in medical research.

Data Cleaning and Preprocessing

Importance of accurate and well-structured information cannot be overstated. This chapter dives into the vital art of data cleaning and preprocessing – a pivotal step in ensuring the data used for medical research and analysis is of the highest quality. We'll explore the techniques and methods that will help you wrangle raw data into a clean, usable format for further analysis.

Healthcare data, by its nature, can be messy. It arrives in various formats, with inconsistencies, missing values, and outliers. This section aims to provide you with a systematic approach to address these issues and prepare your data for insightful analysis.

Techniques for Data Cleaning:

One of the primary tasks in data cleaning is handling missing data. Incomplete records can impede your analysis, making it crucial to decide how to deal with them. Python offers a multitude of tools for this purpose, and libraries like Pandas can be your trusty companions. Here's a code example demonstrating how to handle missing data using Pandas:

```python
import pandas as pd

# Creating a sample DataFrame with missing values
data = {'A': ,
        'B': }
df = pd.DataFrame(data)

# Dropping rows with missing values
df_cleaned = df.dropna()

# Filling missing values with a specific value
df_filled = df.fillna(0)

print("DataFrame with missing values:\n", df)
print("DataFrame after dropping rows with missing values:\n", df_cleaned)
print("DataFrame after filling missing values:\n", df_filled)
```

In the provided Python example, we created a sample DataFrame and then used Pandas to handle missing values. We demonstrated two common techniques: dropping rows with missing values and filling them with a specific value.

Data Preprocessing:

Data preprocessing goes beyond handling missing data. It encompasses a range of activities, such as scaling, encoding categorical data, and feature selection. These processes are essential for creating meaningful insights from your healthcare data.

Take scaling, for instance. Standardizing numerical features can ensure that variables with different ranges do not disproportionately impact the analysis. In the code snippet below, we utilize Scikit-Learn to scale our data:

python

from sklearn.preprocessing import StandardScaler

```
# Create a sample dataset
data = , , , ]
scaler = StandardScaler()

# Fit and transform the data
scaled_data = scaler.fit_transform(data)
```

Scaling data helps maintain consistency and makes it easier to apply various machine learning algorithms.

Feature Selection:

The question of which features are the most relevant for your analysis is often pivotal. Feature selection involves identifying the most influential variables and discarding irrelevant ones. Let's see how you can achieve this using Scikit-Learn:

python

```
from sklearn.feature_selection import SelectKBest
from sklearn.feature_selection import f_regression

# Create a sample dataset with features and target
X = , , ]
y =

# Select top 2 features based on F-regression
selector = SelectKBest(score_func=f_regression, k=2)
X_new = selector.fit_transform(X, y)
```

In this example, we utilized the F-regression method to select the top 2 features. This type of feature selection can significantly impact the performance and efficiency of your analysis.

These are just a few of the techniques you'll encounter when cleaning and preprocessing healthcare data using Python. It's a crucial foundation for the more advanced stages of your data analysis journey. By the time you've completed this section, you'll be well-equipped to whip raw data into shape, ensuring that the insights drawn from it are robust, accurate, and, most importantly, actionable.

Remember, data cleaning and preprocessing are not just about making the data look good. It's about making the data work for you, revealing the hidden gems that can lead to groundbreaking discoveries in the field of healthcare and medical research. In the upcoming chapters, you'll get to apply these cleaned and preprocessed datasets in various analytical and predictive tasks, turning raw information into valuable knowledge.

Merging DataFrames: Bridging the Gap

In healthcare research, data is rarely isolated to a single source. You might have patient records in one DataFrame, lab results in another, and perhaps additional data from external sources. Merging allows you to bring these disparate pieces together, creating a unified dataset for analysis.

One common operation is the 'inner join,' which combines rows from two DataFrames based on a shared key, typically an identifier like patient ID or a timestamp. This operation is useful when you want to retain only the data points that exist in both DataFrames. For example, merging patient records with lab results using a common patient ID can help in associating test results with specific individuals.

```python
import pandas as pd

# Sample DataFrames
patients = pd.DataFrame({'patient_id': ,
                'name': })

lab_results = pd.DataFrame({'patient_id': ,
                'test_result': })

# Inner join on 'patient_id'
```

```
merged_data = pd.merge(patients, lab_results, on='patient_id',
how='inner')
print(merged_data)
```

Output:

```
  patient_id   name test_result
0     2   Bob       85
1     3 Charlie      92
```

This code demonstrates how to merge patient and lab result DataFrames, retaining only the records for patients present in both datasets.

Reshaping Data: A New Perspective

Reshaping data is equally important. There are scenarios in healthcare research where data might be more useful when pivoted or transposed. Pandas provides functions like pivot, melt, and stack that enable you to change the structure of your data, making it more suitable for analysis.

For example, you may have a DataFrame where each row represents a different type of medical measurement, and you want to pivot it to have each measurement type as a column. Here's how you can achieve this:

python

```
# Sample DataFrame
medical_measurements = pd.DataFrame({'patient_id': ,
                        'measurement_type': ,
```

```
                        'value': })
```

```
# Pivot the DataFrame
pivoted_data                                        =
medical_measurements.pivot(index='patient_id',
columns='measurement_type', values='value')
print(pivoted_data)
```

Output:

```
r
```

```
measurement_type  BP  Temperature
patient_id
1               120    NaN
2               NaN    98.6
3               122    NaN
```

In this example, we've pivoted the data, turning different measurement types into columns, making it easier to analyze and compare.

DICOM: Unveiling Medical Images

Picture this: A patient's X-ray, a medical ultrasound, or even a full-fledged MRI scan. These are all vital components of healthcare data, and they typically come in the form of images. To work with these medical images, we turn to DICOM.

What's DICOM?

DICOM is the universal standard for managing, storing, printing, and sharing information in medical imaging. It's the lingua franca of medical imaging data and plays an essential role in healthcare systems worldwide. This format doesn't just contain the image itself; it's enriched with metadata. These data tags are like pieces of a puzzle, describing patient information, the imaging equipment used, and a lot more.

Python in Action: DICOM Handling

Let's say you're building a system to automatically detect anomalies in X-rays. Without the knowledge to handle DICOM files, you're stuck. But with Python's PyDicom library, you're in control. You can read these complex files, extract images, and manipulate metadata effortlessly.

Here's a code snippet:

python

```python
import pydicom

# Load a DICOM file
dicom_file = pydicom.dcmread("your_xray.dcm")

# Extract the patient's name
patient_name = dicom_file.PatientName
print(f"Patient's Name: {patient_name}")

# Access the pixel data
image_data = dicom_file.pixel_array
```

Python, with the PyDicom library, makes it plain sailing to navigate through DICOM files, offering you the power to build sophisticated medical imaging applications.

HL7: Bridging the Gap in Healthcare Data

The healthcare world thrives on data exchange. Patient records, lab results, and billing information must flow seamlessly between different systems. This is where HL7 comes into play.

What's HL7?

Health Level 7 (HL7) is a set of international standards for the transfer of clinical and administrative data between software applications used by various healthcare providers. It ensures that different systems can understand and use the data they receive, facilitating interoperability in healthcare.

Python in Action: HL7 Integration

Let's imagine you're working on a project that involves integrating patient records from a hospital's system into a research database. These records are in HL7 format. Python allows you to parse and process this data with ease.

Here's a code snippet:

python

from hl7 import parser

```
hl7_message          =          "MSH|^~\&|ΛDT1|XYZ|ADT2|ABC|
20220310120030||ADT^A04|6789067|P|2.5"
parsed_message = parser.parse(hl7_message)

# Accessing segments
for segment in parsed_message:
    print(segment)

# Accessing fields within segments
patient_name = parsed_message.segments('PID').field('5')
print(f"Patient Name: {patient_name}")

# Modifying and creating HL7 messages
parsed_message.segments('PID').field('5').value = 'New Name'
new_hl7_message = parsed_message.to_er7()
```

With Python libraries like hl7, you can seamlessly work with HL7 messages. This becomes invaluable in the world of healthcare where data must be understood, exchanged, and utilized with precision.

In essence, Python opens the doors to a realm where healthcare data isn't a mystery. Whether it's intricate DICOM images or the structured language of HL7 messages, Python provides you with the tools and capabilities to make sense of this data. The power of Python in healthcare knows no bounds, and in the upcoming chapters, we'll delve deeper into this fascinating journey. So, let's continue our exploration, shall we?

Summary of Key Concepts

Data handling in healthcare involves various processes, and throughout this chapter, we've delved into the crucial aspects of it. We began by highlighting the significance of proper data handling in healthcare, emphasizing the need for clean, reliable data to draw meaningful insights. Then, we introduced you to the NumPy and Pandas libraries, both indispensable tools for data manipulation in Python.

We explored techniques for cleaning and preprocessing healthcare data, ensuring it's ready for analysis. Understanding how to merge and join DataFrames using Pandas is a fundamental skill, especially when working with diverse datasets. We also touched on the unique data formats often encountered in healthcare, such as DICOM and HL7.

To reinforce these concepts, let's move on to a practical case study that will showcase how these principles can be applied in a real-world scenario.

Case Study: Analyzing Healthcare Data

Scenario:

Imagine you're working for a research institution focused on public health. Your team has gathered a substantial dataset containing information about patients, their medical history, and various health indicators. The goal is to analyze this data and extract insights that can inform public health policies and interventions.

Your Tasks:

1. Data Loading: Start by loading the healthcare dataset. Ensure you're using Pandas for this task.

python

```
import pandas as pd

# Load the dataset
healthcare_data = pd.read_csv('healthcare_data.csv')
```

2. Data Cleaning: Before analysis, check for missing values and outliers in the dataset. Handle them appropriately to maintain data integrity.

python

```
# Check for missing values
missing_values = healthcare_data.isnull().sum()

# Handle missing values
healthcare_data.fillna(method='ffill', inplace=True)  # You can choose your preferred method

# Detect and handle outliers
from scipy import stats
z_scores = stats.zscore(healthcare_data)
healthcare_data = healthcare_data   # You can choose the threshold as per your dataset
```

3. Data Analysis: Utilize Pandas to perform basic statistical analysis on the dataset. Calculate key metrics and visualize relevant data points.

python

```python
# Basic statistics
summary_statistics = healthcare_data.describe()

# Visualize data
import matplotlib.pyplot as plt

# For instance, you can create a histogram of a specific
indicator
plt.hist(healthcare_data, bins=20)
plt.xlabel('Indicator')
plt.ylabel('Frequency')
plt.title('Distribution of Health Indicator')
plt.show()
```

4. Data Interpretation: After performing the analysis, interpret your findings. What do the statistics and visualizations reveal about the health indicators in the dataset? Are there any trends or anomalies that catch your eye?

5. Recommendations: Given your analysis, make data-driven recommendations. For example, if you observe a substantial increase in a specific health indicator in a particular demographic, recommend further investigations and potential public health interventions.

This case study reflects a simplified version of the kind of work you might undertake in healthcare research. It demonstrates how Python, along with the knowledge you've gained in this chapter, can be a powerful tool for extracting valuable insights from healthcare data.

By applying these skills and principles, you'll be better prepared to contribute to the field of healthcare research and make a positive impact on public health. Remember, the key to success in this domain is not just understanding the theory but also applying it to real-world situations.

CHAPTER 4. DATA VISUALIZATION

The ability to effectively communicate data and insights is paramount. This is where data visualization steps into the spotlight. Welcome to the world of turning raw numbers and facts into meaningful, graphical representations that resonate with your audience. In this chapter, we'll embark on a journey through the art and science of data visualization and explore its pivotal role in healthcare data analysis.

Why Data Visualization Matters

You may be wondering why data visualization is such a crucial part of working with healthcare data. The answer is simple yet profound: a well-constructed visual representation can convey complex information in an easily digestible manner. In the context of healthcare, this means that healthcare professionals, researchers, and stakeholders can grasp the intricacies of patient data, medical trends, and clinical outcomes at a glance.

Imagine being able to detect disease outbreaks early by glancing at a map that highlights hotspots of infections. Or picture the impact of showing a graph that visually illustrates how a new treatment is improving patient outcomes over time. These are just a couple of examples of how data visualization can transform the way we analyze and comprehend healthcare data.

Key Concepts in Data Visualization

Before we dive into the practical aspects, it's essential to understand the key concepts of data visualization.

Visual Encoding: This concept involves the use of visual cues to represent data. Things like colors, shapes, sizes, and positions on a chart can all be used to encode different aspects of the data. Effective visual encoding ensures that the viewer can effortlessly interpret the information presented.

Data Types and Appropriate Visuals: Not all data is the same, and different types of data require different visualization techniques. Categorical data, numerical data, time-series data - each needs a specific approach to convey its message effectively.

Perception and Cognition: Understanding how humans perceive and interpret visual information is fundamental. This knowledge helps create visuals that are intuitive and insightful. For instance, we can exploit our ability to quickly spot differences in length to create impactful bar charts.

Storytelling: A good data visualization tells a story. It's not just about displaying numbers; it's about guiding the audience through a narrative. A well-constructed visualization should have a clear message and a call to action.

Python for Data Visualization

In this book, we'll primarily be using Python for data visualization, and the main libraries that will empower us are Matplotlib, Seaborn, and Plotly. Python's versatility and the rich ecosystem of libraries make it an ideal choice for creating visually appealing and informative charts, graphs, and interactive plots.

Matplotlib is a versatile library that provides a solid foundation for creating static, animated, and interactive visualizations in Python. It allows you to build a wide range of charts, from simple line plots to complex heatmaps.

Seaborn, on the other hand, is built on top of Matplotlib and offers a high-level interface for creating aesthetically pleasing statistical graphics. If you want to create sophisticated statistical plots with minimal effort, Seaborn is your go-to tool.

Plotly is perfect for creating interactive visualizations. It enables you to craft dynamic graphs that can be explored and manipulated by s, perfect for building dashboards and reports that convey insights at a glance.

What to Expect

As we delve deeper into this chapter, you can look forward to exploring these libraries in detail. You'll learn how to create various types of charts, enhance their aesthetics, and tell compelling data-driven stories.

Whether you're a healthcare professional seeking to present patient data effectively or a researcher aiming to communicate findings to a broader audience, mastering data visualization is a critical skill. So, let's embark on this journey, armed with Python and the tools to make healthcare data come to life through the magic of visualization. In the following sections, we'll explore Matplotlib, Seaborn, and Plotly in depth, providing you with the knowledge and techniques needed to bring data to life in the world of healthcare and medical research.

For now, let's start our exploration of Matplotlib, the fundamental library for data visualization in Python. In the subsection that follows, we'll dive into the basics and create our first Python visualization.

Example of Data Visualization using Matplotlib

Now that we've grasped the importance of data visualization and its key concepts, it's time to roll up our sleeves and start creating visualizations using Matplotlib, one of the core libraries for data visualization in Python.

Consider this scenario: You're a healthcare researcher examining the monthly patient admission rates at your hospital. To better understand the trends, you decide to visualize this data. Here's how you can do it using Python and Matplotlib.

Let's start by assuming you have the following data:

python

```
# Sample data
months =
admission_rates =
```

With this data, we can create a simple line plot using Matplotlib. This will allow you to visualize how patient admission rates have fluctuated over the first six months of the year.

python

```
import matplotlib.pyplot as plt

# Create a line plot
plt.plot(months, admission_rates, marker='o', linestyle='-')

# Adding labels and title
plt.xlabel('Months')
plt.ylabel('Admission Rates')
plt.title('Monthly Patient Admission Rates in 2023')

# Display the plot
plt.show()
```

In this example, we used Matplotlib to create a line plot. The plot function is used to generate the actual graph, and xlabel, ylabel, and title functions help to label and title the plot.

This is just a glimpse of what Matplotlib can do. In the upcoming sections, we'll explore more types of visualizations, customization options, and real-world healthcare data scenarios to strengthen your data visualization skills.

The ability to transform raw data into meaningful visuals is a powerful skill in healthcare and medical research. As we progress through this chapter, you'll not only understand the mechanics of creating visualizations but also master the art of telling compelling stories with your data.

findings effectively.

Matplotlib's Introduction:

Matplotlib, as the name suggests, is your passport to creating captivating visual plots, charts, and graphs. With a rich assortment of features, this library empowers you to construct visually appealing representations of healthcare data, such as patient statistics, clinical trends, and research results. The - friendly nature of Matplotlib allows you to get started with plotting swiftly, whether you're a beginner or an experienced Python enthusiast.

Visualizing Health Data:

Before we delve into the nuts and bolts of Matplotlib, it's crucial to understand the significance of data visualization in healthcare. In a field where every data point can impact patient well-being, healthcare professionals, researchers, and analysts must present their findings in a comprehensible and impactful manner. Matplotlib aids in this endeavor by offering a vast array of chart types, from simple line graphs to complex heatmaps.

Let's consider a hypothetical scenario to illustrate the power of Matplotlib. Imagine you're working on a research project involving patient cholesterol levels over time. With Matplotlib, you can effortlessly create line plots that display how cholesterol levels change for different patients or age groups. These visualizations can help identify trends, outliers, or potential areas for further investigation.

Getting Started with Matplotlib:

To start using Matplotlib for your healthcare data visualization needs, you need to import the library into your Python environment. Here's a simple example to kickstart your journey:

```python
import matplotlib.pyplot as plt

# Sample data - patient age vs. cholesterol level
patient_age =
cholesterol_level =

# Create a line plot
plt.plot(patient_age, cholesterol_level, marker='o', linestyle='-', color='b', label='Cholesterol Level')
plt.xlabel('Patient Age')
plt.ylabel('Cholesterol Level (mg/dL)')
plt.title('Cholesterol Levels Over Age')
plt.legend()
plt.grid(True)

# Display the plot
plt.show()
```

In this example, we import Matplotlib and use it to create a basic line plot showcasing the relationship between patient age and cholesterol levels. We customize the plot by specifying markers, line styles, colors, labels, and titles, which can be tailored to your specific healthcare data.

Matplotlib's versatility allows you to experiment with various plot types, like bar charts, scatter plots, histograms, and more, to bring out the most critical aspects of your healthcare data.

Furthermore, as you progress in your healthcare data visualization journey, you'll learn to leverage Matplotlib's advanced features, including customizing aesthetics, incorporating multiple plots, and creating interactive visualizations for more in-depth exploration of your medical research data.

By mastering Matplotlib, you'll unlock the ability to communicate your findings effectively, enabling fellow healthcare professionals, researchers, and stakeholders to comprehend the insights drawn from your Python-powered data analysis. Whether you're examining patient records, clinical trials, or public health data, Matplotlib will prove to be an invaluable companion on your journey toward better healthcare outcomes.

Seaborn for Statistical Plots

Seaborn, a data visualization library built on top of Matplotlib, is designed to create beautiful, concise, and informative statistical graphics. Its ease of use and aesthetic appeal make it a valuable asset for anyone diving into healthcare data analysis.

Why Seaborn?

Before we delve into the practical aspects of Seaborn, let's understand why it's worth exploring. Seaborn's primary strength lies in its ability to simplify complex data visualizations. It excels in:

Statistical Plots: Seaborn specializes in creating a wide range of statistical plots. These visuals go beyond basic bar charts and scatter plots, enabling you to explore relationships, distributions, and patterns within your healthcare data.

Integration with Pandas: Seaborn seamlessly integrates with Pandas DataFrames. This means that you can easily work with your healthcare datasets, apply statistical functions, and plot the results using Seaborn.

Aesthetics: Seaborn offers visually pleasing default themes and color palettes, ensuring that your plots are not only informative but also attractive. You can impress your audience with clear, vibrant visuals.

Exploring Seaborn in Practice

Let's embark on a journey into the world of Seaborn by exploring some common statistical plots and how to create them. Remember that the best way to learn is by doing, so if you have Python installed, you can follow along.

Note: If you haven't installed Seaborn, you can do so using pip:

python

pip install seaborn

Example 1: Box Plots

Box plots are fantastic for visualizing the distribution of data.

They display the median, quartiles, and potential outliers in your dataset. Here's how you can create a box plot using Seaborn:

python

```
import seaborn as sns
import matplotlib.pyplot as plt

# Assuming 'data' is your healthcare dataset
sns.set(style="whitegrid") # Set the style
plt.figure(figsize=(10, 6)) # Set the figure size

# Create a box plot for a specific column
sns.boxplot(x=data)

# Adding labels and title
plt.xlabel("Age")
plt.title("Distribution of Age in Healthcare Data")

plt.show()
```

Example 2: Pair Plots

Pair plots are incredibly useful when you want to visualize relationships between multiple variables. Seaborn makes it effortless to create them:

python

```
# Assuming 'data' is your healthcare dataset
```

```
sns.set(style="ticks")  # Set the style
sns.pairplot(data, hue="smoker")

plt.show()
```

Example 3: Heatmaps

Heatmaps are excellent for showing correlations between variables. In healthcare, this can be crucial. Let's create a simple heatmap:

python

```
# Assuming 'data' is your healthcare dataset
correlation_matrix = data.corr()

plt.figure(figsize=(10, 8))
sns.heatmap(correlation_matrix,                    annot=True,
cmap="coolwarm")

plt.title("Correlation Heatmap for Healthcare Data")
plt.show()
```

In Closing

Seaborn offers a plethora of other statistical plots, such as violin plots, regression plots, and count plots, each serving a specific analytical purpose. As you venture further into the world of healthcare data analysis, mastering Seaborn will empower you to extract meaningful insights and communicate them effectively.

Remember that the key to becoming proficient with Seaborn, as with any tool, is practice. Experiment with different types of plots, apply them to your healthcare data, and don't hesitate to tweak the aesthetics to make your visualizations more engaging. The fusion of Python, Seaborn, and healthcare data has the potential to uncover valuable insights and drive innovations in the medical field.

So, roll up your sleeves, open your Jupyter Notebook, and let Seaborn guide you through the intricate realm of statistical plots in healthcare data analysis. Your journey into the world of advanced visualizations begins now.

Customization

Customization is key when it comes to conveying your data's message effectively. To create compelling visualizations, it's essential to tailor them to your audience and the specific data you're working with. Python, with its versatile libraries like Matplotlib, Seaborn, and Plotly, offers you a wide range of options to customize your visualizations.

Customizing Aesthetics:

Visualizations should be aesthetically pleasing while ensuring clarity. You can customize colors, fonts, markers, and line styles to match the overall theme of your project or organization. For instance, Matplotlib allows you to set custom colors and styles to make your plots visually consistent. Here's an example:

python

```python
import matplotlib.pyplot as plt

# Customize line style, color, and marker
plt.plot(x, y, linestyle='--', color='blue', marker='o',
markersize=8, label='Data Points')

# Set labels and title
plt.xlabel('X-axis')
plt.ylabel('Y-axis')
plt.title('Customized Line Plot')

# Add a legend
plt.legend()
plt.show()
```

Enhancing Interactivity:

In the age of interactive data exploration, enhancing your visualizations with interactive features is crucial. Plotly, a popular library, enables you to create interactive charts that allow s to zoom, pan, and explore data points. Here's an example of an interactive scatter plot:

python

```python
import plotly.express as px

# Create an interactive scatter plot
fig = px.scatter(data_frame, x='X-axis', y='Y-axis',
color='Category', title='Interactive Scatter Plot')
```

```
# Customize the layout
fig.update_layout(
    xaxis_title='X-axis',
    yaxis_title='Y-axis',
    legend_title='Category',
    hovermode='closest'
)

fig.show()
```

Adding Annotations and Text:

Annotations and text play a vital role in highlighting specific data points or trends. You can add annotations to your visualizations using functions provided by Matplotlib. For instance, you can annotate a data point like this:

python

```
# Annotate a specific data point
plt.annotate('Max Value', xy=(x_max, y_max), xytext=(x_max - 5, y_max + 10),
        arrowprops=dict(arrowstyle='->',
connectionstyle='arc3,rad=0.5'))
```

Customizing Axes and Grids:

Customizing axes and grids can significantly improve the clarity of your visualizations. You can control axis labels, ticks, and gridlines in Matplotlib. For example:

python

```python
# Customize axis labels and ticks
plt.xticks(range(1, 6), )
plt.yticks()
```

```python
# Add gridlines
plt.grid(True, linestyle='--', alpha=0.7)
```

Combining Multiple Visualizations:

Sometimes, combining different plots can provide a more comprehensive view of the data. You can create subplots and overlays using Matplotlib to achieve this. Here's an example of combining a bar chart and a line chart:

python

```python
# Create subplots
fig, ax1 = plt.subplots()
```

```python
# Create bar chart on the first subplot
ax1.bar(x, bar_data, color='b', alpha=0.7, label='Bars')
ax1.set_xlabel('X-axis')
ax1.set_ylabel('Bars')
```

```python
# Create a line chart on the second subplot
ax2 = ax1.twinx()
ax2.plot(x, line_data, color='r', linestyle='--', marker='o',
```

```
label='Line')
ax2.set_ylabel('Line')

# Add legends for both plots
fig.legend(loc='upper left')
plt.show()
```

Customizing and enhancing your visualizations is all about making your data tell a compelling story. Whether it's adjusting the aesthetics, adding interactivity, or combining different visual elements, Python's libraries provide you with the tools you need to create powerful and engaging data representations. Keep in mind that the best visualizations are not only informative but also visually captivating, ensuring your audience can easily grasp the insights you want to convey.

Visualizing Healthcare Data

Welcome to the exciting world of data visualization in the realm of healthcare. In this section, we will explore the art and science of presenting healthcare data in a visually compelling and informative manner. Data visualization is a powerful tool that allows healthcare professionals, researchers, and decision-makers to gain insights, identify trends, and communicate findings effectively.

The Power of Visuals

Before we dive into the practical aspects, let's reflect on why data visualization matters in healthcare. The human brain is wired to process visual information much more efficiently than raw numbers or text. Visualizations can transform complex datasets into understandable patterns, making it easier to make informed decisions and convey critical information to stakeholders.

Selecting the Right Visualization

One of the first considerations when visualizing healthcare data is choosing the right type of visualization. The choice depends on the nature of the data and the insights you aim to convey. Some common types of healthcare data visualizations include:

Line Charts: Ideal for showing trends over time, such as patient vital signs or disease prevalence.

Bar Charts: Useful for comparisons, such as hospital performance metrics or medication effectiveness.

Pie Charts: Suitable for displaying parts of a whole, such as the distribution of different diseases in a population.

Scatter Plots: Great for identifying relationships between two variables, like the correlation between body mass index and blood pressure.

Heatmaps: Effective for visualizing variations in data, such as the geographic distribution of disease outbreaks.

Interactive Dashboards: These allow s to explore data on their terms, which is invaluable for decision-making.

Python for Healthcare Data Visualization

Now, let's get hands-on and explore how Python can be your trusted companion for creating stunning healthcare data visualizations. Python offers a range of libraries for this purpose, with Matplotlib, Seaborn, and Plotly being some of the most popular choices. Here, we'll use Matplotlib as an example to illustrate the power of Python.

python

```
# Importing Matplotlib library
import matplotlib.pyplot as plt

# Sample data
months =
patient_count =

# Creating a simple bar chart
plt.bar(months, patient_count, color='skyblue')
plt.title('Monthly Patient Count')
plt.xlabel('Months')
plt.ylabel('Number of Patients')
plt.show()
```

In the Python code snippet above, we import the Matplotlib library and create a basic bar chart showing the monthly patient count. This is just a glimpse of what Python is capable of in terms of healthcare data visualization.

Customization and Enhancement

A key advantage of using Python for healthcare data visualization is the flexibility it offers. You can customize and enhance your visualizations to meet your specific needs. Whether it's adjusting colors, adding labels, or highlighting specific data points, Python gives you the tools to make your visualizations both informative and visually appealing.

Interactive Visualizations with Plotly

Python's Plotly library takes healthcare data visualization a step further by allowing you to create interactive charts and dashboards. This is particularly useful when dealing with large healthcare datasets or when you want to empower end-s to explore data on their own.

Here's a simple example of creating an interactive line chart with Plotly:

python

```
# Importing Plotly library
import plotly.express as px

# Sample data
months =
patient_count =

# Creating an interactive line chart
fig = px.line(x=months, y=patient_count, title='Monthly Patient Count')
fig.update_xaxes(title_text='Months')
```

fig.update_yaxes(title_text='Number of Patients')

fig.show()

This code snippet illustrates how to use Plotly to create an interactive line chart to display monthly patient counts.

In this section, we've explored the significance of data visualization in healthcare and the power of Python in this domain. Python, with its libraries like Matplotlib and Plotly, equips you with the tools needed to bring healthcare data to life, making it accessible and actionable. Whether you're tracking patient outcomes, monitoring the spread of diseases, or evaluating the performance of healthcare facilities, data visualization is your ally in transforming raw data into valuable insights. As you delve deeper into the world of healthcare data analysis, remember that data visualization is not just about making data look good; it's about making data tell meaningful stories.

Interactive Data Visualization with Plotly

Data visualization is an essential tool for understanding complex healthcare data, and Plotly takes it to the next level by allowing you to create interactive and dynamic charts and graphs. It's not just about presenting data; it's about engaging your audience, providing them with the means to explore and comprehend information intuitively.

One of the outstanding features of Plotly is its ability to generate interactive visualizations with ease. This section will guide you through the process of integrating Plotly into your Python toolkit and leveraging it for healthcare data visualization. We'll explore the various chart types, how to customize them, and the best practices for creating compelling visuals.

Let's start with a basic example of an interactive Plotly chart:

python

```python
import plotly.express as px
import pandas as pd

# Create a sample dataset
data = pd.DataFrame({
    'Month': ,
    'Patients':
})

# Create an interactive bar chart
fig = px.bar(data, x='Month', y='Patients', title='Monthly Patient Count')
fig.update_xaxes(title_text='Month')
fig.update_yaxes(title_text='Number of Patients')
fig.show()
```

In this code, we first import the necessary libraries, including Plotly and Pandas. Then, we create a sample dataset and use Plotly to generate an interactive bar chart displaying the monthly patient count. s can hover over the bars to see precise values, zoom in, pan, and even export the chart. This level of interactivity can significantly enhance data exploration.

Why Choose Plotly for Healthcare Data Visualization?

Plotly's interactivity isn't limited to bar charts; you can create line charts, scatter plots, pie charts, and much more. This versatility makes it ideal for visualizing diverse healthcare data, from patient demographics to clinical trial results.

Moreover, when dealing with large datasets, interactive features become indispensable. Plotly allows you to handle and present extensive data in an easily digestible manner. s can filter, drill down, and explore the data points that interest them the most.

Imagine creating an interactive heatmap that showcases disease prevalence across geographic regions, enabling researchers and healthcare professionals to identify areas with the highest need for specific medical interventions. With Plotly, this is not only possible but also highly effective.

To fully harness the potential of Plotly, it's essential to understand its capabilities and customization options. This section delves into the details, explaining how to configure Plotly charts, add interactivity, and tailor the visualizations to your specific needs. You'll learn how to create interactive dashboards and reports that provide valuable insights into healthcare trends and patterns.

As we delve deeper into this subsection, you'll come across more intricate examples and case studies that demonstrate how Plotly can be applied to real-world healthcare scenarios. Whether you're analyzing patient outcomes, clinical trial data, or health system performance, Plotly's interactive features will prove invaluable.

So, get ready to embark on a journey through the world of

interactive data visualization with Plotly. This section will equip you with the knowledge and skills needed to create captivating visualizations that facilitate healthcare research, decision-making, and innovation. With each chart you build, you'll be one step closer to unlocking the potential of Python in healthcare and medical research.

Remember, data visualization is not just about displaying data; it's about telling a story. Plotly is your pen, and your healthcare data is the canvas. Let's paint a compelling narrative together.

Case Studies in Data Visualization

Welcome to an exciting journey through real-world applications of data visualization in healthcare. In this section, we will explore practical case studies that highlight the power of Python in transforming complex healthcare data into insightful visual representations. These case studies serve as windows into the diverse and impactful ways data visualization contributes to medical research and patient care.

Case Study 1: Monitoring Disease Trends

Imagine you're a public health analyst working on tracking disease trends in a particular region. Your task is to gather and analyze healthcare data to monitor the prevalence of a disease. Python's data visualization libraries, such as Matplotlib and Seaborn, offer a dynamic toolkit for this purpose.

In this case study, we'll dive into the process of visualizing disease spread over time. We'll use Python to create interactive line charts, heatmaps, and geographic plots, allowing us to detect outbreaks and study the impact of interventions. With Python's tools, you can craft visually appealing and informative representations of complex health data.

Case Study 2: Clinical Trial Outcomes

Clinical trials are at the heart of medical research, and understanding their outcomes is crucial. Python's data visualization capabilities come into play by helping researchers and clinicians comprehend vast amounts of clinical trial data.

In this case study, we'll explore how Python can be used to visualize the efficacy of new drugs or treatments. By creating bar charts, scatter plots, and forest plots, we can visually compare treatment groups, identify trends, and uncover any adverse effects. Python empowers researchers to make data-driven decisions by providing clear insights into clinical trial results.

Case Study 3: Radiological Imaging Analysis

Medical imaging, such as X-rays, MRIs, and CT scans, generates enormous datasets that demand efficient visualization techniques. Python's libraries, combined with deep learning, enable us to unlock the full potential of radiological images.

In this case study, we'll delve into the realm of radiology and demonstrate how Python can be used to enhance medical image analysis. We'll use Convolutional Neural Networks (CNNs) to classify images, and Matplotlib to visualize the results. Additionally, we'll showcase how interactive visualizations can assist radiologists in making accurate diagnoses. Python's deep learning capabilities combined with data visualization revolutionize the field of medical imaging.

Case Study 4: Predictive Analytics for Patient Outcomes

Predictive analytics play a vital role in healthcare, helping providers anticipate patient outcomes and allocate resources effectively. Python, with its data visualization libraries, facilitates predictive modeling and provides valuable insights into patient care.

In this case study, we'll see how Python can predict patient outcomes based on various factors, such as demographics, medical history, and treatment plans. We'll use Python's machine learning capabilities to build predictive models and then create intuitive dashboards using Plotly. These dashboards allow healthcare professionals to interact with the data, adjust parameters, and gain a better understanding of the risks and potential interventions.

Case Study 5: Tracking Public Health Indicators

Public health officials rely on data to make informed decisions and take actions to protect communities. Python's data visualization capabilities come to the rescue in visualizing and tracking public health indicators.

In this case study, we'll explore the visualization of public health data, such as vaccination rates, disease outbreaks, and environmental factors. Python enables us to create choropleth maps, animated graphs, and dashboards that display real-time data. By understanding these visualizations, public health officials can make timely interventions and policies to safeguard the well-being of the population.

By delving into these practical case studies, you'll witness firsthand how Python transforms raw healthcare data into actionable insights. The visualizations we create will empower healthcare professionals, researchers, and analysts to make informed decisions, leading to better patient care and significant advancements in the field of medical research.

In the following Python code snippets, we will demonstrate the key components of each case study. These examples will provide you with a hands-on understanding of how Python can be used for data visualization in healthcare. Whether you're an aspiring data scientist, a healthcare professional, or simply curious about the intersection of Python and healthcare, these case studies will inspire you to explore the endless possibilities this dynamic duo offers.

Let's embark on this exciting journey, using Python to unveil the hidden stories within healthcare data through the art of data visualization.

The Power of Visualizing Healthcare Data

Our exploration began with an understanding of the significance of data visualization in the healthcare domain. Visual representations of medical data are not just aesthetically pleasing; they provide a clear and concise means of conveying information. These visualizations help healthcare professionals, researchers, and decision-makers grasp complex patterns, trends, and anomalies, thereby driving informed decisions and better patient outcomes.

Matplotlib and Seaborn: Tools for the Trade:

In the realm of Python libraries, Matplotlib and Seaborn emerged as our trusted companions for crafting data visualizations. Matplotlib, with its flexibility, empowers you to create a wide array of basic plots, while Seaborn brings forth the capabilities for crafting advanced and statistically meaningful visualizations. These tools, combined, provide you with the arsenal to represent healthcare data in compelling ways.

Customization and Enhancement:

In the world of data visualization, aesthetics matter. You've learned how to tailor your visualizations to meet specific needs and objectives. Whether it's adding labels, colors, or incorporating interactive elements, Python offers you the flexibility to customize your charts and graphs. Aesthetically pleasing visuals not only make your findings more engaging but also enhance their communicative power.

Realizing the Potential: Healthcare Data Visualization:

As we ventured deeper into the chapter, you've seen healthcare data come to life. From plotting patient vital signs over time to analyzing population health trends, you now possess the skills to turn raw data into actionable insights. This capacity is invaluable in myriad scenarios, ranging from monitoring patient progress to tracking the spread of diseases.

Plotly: Bridging the Gap to Interactivity:

In today's data-driven world, the ability to create interactive data visualizations has become a highly sought-after skill. Plotly, our chosen tool for this purpose, lets you craft dashboards and interactive charts with ease. These dynamic visualizations not only engage your audience but also allow them to explore data on their own terms.

Case Studies: Bridging Theory and Practice:

Real-world application is the touchstone of knowledge. The chapter brought you practical case studies, each showcasing the power of data visualization in healthcare. From tracking the progress of an epidemic to monitoring patient vital signs, these cases have illuminated the real-life applications of the concepts you've learned.

Key Takeaways:

Visual Storytelling: Data visualization is not just about graphs and charts; it's a medium for telling compelling stories with data.

Matplotlib and Seaborn: Two powerful Python libraries that cater to different aspects of data visualization.

Customization is Key: The ability to customize and enhance visualizations adds a layer of professionalism to your work.

Interactivity Matters: Interactive visualizations provide a richer experience and deeper engagement.

Practice Makes Perfect: The case studies demonstrate that practical experience is where your newfound skills truly shine.

CHAPTER 5. DATA PREPROCESSING

Imagine a dataset that's riddled with missing values, outliers, or inconsistencies. Without proper preprocessing, the analysis performed on such data could lead to incorrect diagnoses, skewed research findings, or even decisions detrimental to patient care. Data preprocessing is the remedy that ensures data quality and integrity, setting the stage for reliable analysis.

The significance of data preprocessing in healthcare cannot be overstated. It helps in:

1. Data Cleaning: This is the process of handling missing values, correcting errors, and ensuring the dataset is complete. In the healthcare domain, where data accuracy is paramount, addressing missing or erroneous entries can be a matter of life and death.

2. Outlier Detection and Treatment: Outliers, data points significantly different from the majority, can distort statistical analysis. Detecting and handling outliers is vital, as they could represent critical medical cases or anomalies in research data.

3. Scaling and Normalization: Healthcare data can encompass measurements from diverse scales and units. Scaling and

normalization make sure that these variations don't unduly influence the analysis.

4. Encoding Categorical Data: Patient data often includes categorical variables like blood types, diseases, or medication names. Converting these variables into a numerical format is essential for machine learning algorithms.

5. Feature Selection: The feature selection process entails identifying the most relevant attributes or variables for a particular analysis, thereby reducing complexity and increasing efficiency.

By addressing these aspects and more, data preprocessing ensures that healthcare professionals and researchers can rely on the data's quality and accuracy for their critical work.

Python's Role in Data Preprocessing

Now, let's talk about the Pythonic approach to data preprocessing. Python provides a myriad of libraries and tools that make the process efficient and effective. Whether you're working with electronic health records (EHRs), clinical trial data, medical imaging, or patient records, Python offers versatile solutions.

One of the primary libraries that stand out in this context is Pandas. Pandas provides an extensive toolkit for data manipulation, including functionalities for handling missing data, dealing with outliers, and performing data transformations. The code example below illustrates how Pandas can help address missing data:

python

```
import pandas as pd

# Load healthcare data into a Pandas DataFrame
healthcare_data = pd.read_csv('healthcare_data.csv')

# Check for missing values
missing_values = healthcare_data.isnull().sum()

# Fill missing values with the mean of the respective column
healthcare_data.fillna(healthcare_data.mean(), inplace=True)
```

In this example, we use Pandas to load a healthcare dataset, identify missing values, and fill them with the mean value of their respective columns. This is just a glimpse of how Python can facilitate data preprocessing in healthcare.

As we delve deeper into the intricacies of data preprocessing in the subsequent sections, you'll discover more Pythonic solutions and gain a comprehensive understanding of how to prepare healthcare data for accurate and insightful analysis. Whether you're a healthcare professional, a researcher, or an aspiring data scientist, this chapter will equip you with the knowledge and tools necessary to harness the potential of healthcare data through Python.

So, fasten your seatbelts and get ready to embark on a journey through the world of data preprocessing in healthcare with Python as your trusty companion. With each section, you'll uncover new techniques, methods, and Python code snippets to master this indispensable phase of the data analysis process.

Handling Missing Data

Handling missing data in healthcare datasets is a critical aspect of data preprocessing. In the real world, data is rarely perfect, and gaps or missing values are commonplace. In this section, we will explore various strategies and techniques to effectively manage missing data, ensuring the integrity and reliability of your healthcare dataset.

Identifying Missing Data:

Before we delve into strategies, it's essential to identify and understand the nature of missing data in your dataset. Missing data can take different forms:

Missing Completely at Random (MCAR): This type of missing data occurs when the missingness is unrelated to any other variable in the dataset. It's a random occurrence, and there's no pattern to it.

Missing at Random (MAR): Missingness depends on other variables in the dataset, but not on the variable with missing data. For example, if a questionnaire is missed by younger patients, this could be considered MAR.

Missing Not at Random (MNAR): In this case, the missingness depends on the value of the variable itself. For instance, if patients with higher cholesterol levels are less likely to report their cholesterol readings, it's MNAR.

Strategies for Handling Missing Data:

Deletion: The simplest strategy is to remove rows or columns with missing data. While this might be suitable for MCAR data, it can result in significant information loss.

Imputation: Imputation involves estimating or filling in missing values. Common methods include mean, median, or mode imputation, where you replace missing values with the mean (average), median (middle value), or mode (most frequent value) of the variable. More advanced techniques include regression imputation, where you predict missing values based on other variables.

Multiple Imputation: This method creates multiple imputed datasets and analyzes them separately, then combines the results. Multiple imputation accounts for the uncertainty in imputed values and often provides more accurate results.

Advanced Techniques: Machine learning models can be used for imputation. For instance, you can train a model to predict missing values based on other features in the dataset. This approach can be especially useful when dealing with MNAR data.

Python Code Example:

Let's illustrate a simple imputation technique using Python. We'll impute missing values in a pandas DataFrame using the mean imputation method.

python

```
import pandas as pd
```

```
# Assuming 'df' is your DataFrame with missing data
# Impute missing values with the mean of the column
df.fillna(df.mean(), inplace=True)
```

In this example, 'missing_column' represents the column with missing data. We replace the missing values with the mean of that column. You can adapt this code to your specific dataset and imputation method.

Handling missing data in healthcare datasets is crucial to ensure the accuracy and reliability of your analyses. Identifying the type of missingness and selecting the appropriate strategy is essential. Python, with its rich ecosystem of libraries like pandas, offers a wide range of tools to effectively manage missing data. Imputation methods can vary depending on the nature of your dataset, and choosing the right technique is essential for sound analysis and decision-making in healthcare research.

Outlier Detection and Treatment

Before we embark on the journey of treating outliers, we must first identify them. Python offers several libraries and techniques to help us with this crucial step. One of the most common methods is the use of box plots. Box plots provide a visual representation of the data's distribution, making outliers more apparent. We can use the seaborn library, introduced earlier in this book, to create insightful box plots.

Here's an example of how you can create a box plot to identify outliers in a dataset:

python

```
import seaborn as sns
import matplotlib.pyplot as plt

# Assuming 'data' is your dataset
sns.set(style="whitegrid")
plt.figure(figsize=(8, 6))
sns.boxplot(x=data)
plt.title("Box Plot for Outlier Detection")
plt.show()
```

The box plot will clearly display any data points that fall outside the whiskers, indicating potential outliers.

Treating Outliers

Once we've identified the outliers, the next step is to decide how to handle them. There are various strategies we can employ, and the choice often depends on the specific characteristics of the data and the goals of the analysis.

   Removal: The simplest approach is to remove the outliers from the dataset. This can be done using conditional indexing. For instance:

python

```
# Assuming 'data' is your dataset
data = data < upper_threshold]
```

Transformation: In some cases, transforming the data can help mitigate the impact of outliers. Common transformations include the logarithmic or square root transformation.

Winsorization: This technique involves replacing extreme values with values that are closer to the mean or median. For instance:

python

from scipy.stats.mstats import winsorize

# Winsorize the data between the 5th and 95th percentiles
data = winsorize(data, limits=)

Imputation: For certain datasets, it may be more appropriate to impute the outliers with estimated values, rather than remove them. You can use statistical methods or machine learning models to impute missing or outlier values.

Robust Statistical Methods: Consider using statistical methods that are less sensitive to outliers, such as the median and percentile-based statistics, instead of the mean.

Each of these strategies has its pros and cons, and your choice will depend on the specific context of your analysis.

It's important to mention that outlier detection and treatment are not isolated tasks. They should be part of a broader data preprocessing pipeline, which includes handling missing values, scaling, and encoding categorical data, as we discussed in earlier sections of this book.

Identifying and handling outliers in healthcare data is a vital step to ensure the accuracy and reliability of your analyses. Python, with its versatile libraries and tools, equips you to tackle this task efficiently. Always remember that the approach you choose should align with the nature of your data and the objectives of your analysis. Whether you're conducting research on patient outcomes or studying medical trends, your ability to manage outliers effectively will contribute to the quality and validity of your findings.

In the next section, we'll delve into another aspect of data preprocessing: scaling and normalization. These techniques play a crucial role in preparing healthcare data for various analyses and machine learning applications.

Scaling and Normalization

In the realm of healthcare data analysis, we often encounter datasets with varying ranges and units. These inconsistencies can pose significant challenges when applying machine learning algorithms, as they might prioritize one feature over another due to their inherent differences. This is where the crucial concepts of scaling and normalization come into play, ensuring that our data is on a level playing field.

Scaling for Consistency

Imagine you have a healthcare dataset that includes a patient's age, blood pressure, and cholesterol levels. The age might be in the range of 0-100 years, while blood pressure ranges from 60-200 mmHg, and cholesterol values can span 100-300 mg/dL. Machine learning algorithms often rely on the concept of distances between data points. If we don't scale these features, the algorithm might heavily favor attributes with larger numerical values, potentially leading to skewed results.

Scaling involves transforming your data into a common range, often between 0 and 1 or -1 and 1. This equalizes the importance of each feature. Let's consider an example in Python:

python

from sklearn.preprocessing import MinMaxScaler

# Create a Min-Max scaler
scaler = MinMaxScaler()

# Scaling the age, blood pressure, and cholesterol columns
data] = scaler.fit_transform(data])

Here, the MinMaxScaler scales the specified columns to values between 0 and 1. This process ensures that the age, blood pressure, and cholesterol features are equally influential during machine learning model training.

Normalization for Uniformity

Normalization goes one step further, focusing on the distribution of data points within a single feature. It aims to make the data conform to a normal (Gaussian) distribution with a mean of 0 and a standard deviation of 1. Normalization is particularly useful when dealing with models that assume a Gaussian distribution of the features.

Suppose you're working with a dataset containing patient weights. Some weights might be measured in pounds, while others are in kilograms. To ensure uniformity and comparability, you would normalize the data.

Let's use Python to illustrate this process:

python

```
from sklearn.preprocessing import StandardScaler

# Create a StandardScaler
scaler = StandardScaler()

# Normalize the weight column
data = scaler.fit_transform(data])
```

In this example, the StandardScaler transforms the 'weight' column to have a mean of 0 and a standard deviation of 1. This standardization simplifies the interpretation of coefficients in linear models and aids in achieving better convergence during training.

By incorporating scaling and normalization techniques, we ensure that our healthcare data is well-prepared for analysis and modeling. These practices help data scientists and healthcare professionals obtain more accurate and meaningful insights, ultimately contributing to better decision-making in patient care and medical research.

Understanding Categorical Data

Before we dive into the technical aspects of handling categorical data, it's essential to grasp the significance of this data type in healthcare. Categorical data provides valuable information for patient demographics, diagnoses, and medical specialties. It allows us to group, label, and organize data, making it easier to interpret and analyze.

In Python, we typically use libraries such as Pandas for this purpose. Let's start by importing the necessary libraries and setting up our environment:

python

```
import pandas as pd
```

Now, imagine we have a dataset containing patient information, and one of the columns is "Gender." It might look like this:

python

```
data = {
    'PatientID': ,
    'Gender':
}

df = pd.DataFrame(data)
```

Label Encoding

One way to handle categorical data is through label encoding.

This method assigns a unique numerical label to each category. For instance, 'Male' could be encoded as 0, 'Female' as 1, and 'Other' as 2. This transformation can be achieved using Scikit-Learn:

python

```
from sklearn.preprocessing import LabelEncoder
```

```
label_encoder = LabelEncoder()
df = label_encoder.fit_transform(df)
```

Label encoding is a simple and efficient technique, especially when dealing with binary categories. However, it may introduce unintended ordinal relationships between the categories, which can be misleading.

One-Hot Encoding

To avoid the issues associated with label encoding, we can turn to one-hot encoding. This method creates binary columns for each category, indicating its presence with a 1 or 0. Let's apply one-hot encoding to our 'Gender' column:

python

```
df = pd.get_dummies(df, columns=, prefix=)
```

Now, our DataFrame looks like this:

python

PatientID	Gender_Encoded	Gender_Female	Gender_Male	Gender_Other
0	1	1	1	0	0
1	2	0	0	1	0
2	3	1	1	0	0
3	4	2	0	0	1
4	5	0	0	1	0

When to Use Which

The choice between label encoding and one-hot encoding depends on the nature of your categorical data and the machine learning algorithm you intend to use. Label encoding is suitable when there's an inherent order or relationship between the categories. For example, in a dataset where categories represent education levels, 'High School' is lower than 'Bachelor's Degree.'

On the other hand, one-hot encoding is a safer choice when categories are nominal, with no implied order. It's also preferred for algorithms that might misinterpret ordinal relationships as meaningful.

In healthcare data analysis, you'll frequently encounter categorical data in the form of medical specialties, medications, or patient conditions. Properly handling this data ensures that your models receive accurate input, contributing to more precise and reliable results.

In the next section, we'll explore the critical process of feature selection, highlighting methods to choose the most relevant variables for medical data analysis.

Feature Selection

In the realm of healthcare and medical research, data can be overwhelmingly abundant. While having access to a vast amount of data can be a boon, it can also be a bane if not efficiently managed. Feature selection emerges as a critical step in the data preprocessing pipeline. This process is akin to a diligent curator, carefully selecting the most valuable pieces for an exhibition, ensuring that they represent the essence of the entire collection. In this section, we will delve into the art of feature selection, its significance, and some Python-based techniques that make this process more efficient.

The Significance of Feature Selection

Imagine you're dealing with a healthcare dataset that contains numerous attributes or features, such as patient demographics, medical history, lab results, and more. While it might seem beneficial to use all of this information for analysis, including irrelevant or redundant features can lead to several problems. These may include overfitting, increased computational complexity, and decreased model interpretability. In essence, too many features can obscure the signal within the data, making it difficult to extract meaningful insights.

Feature selection addresses this issue by identifying and retaining only the most informative and relevant attributes. This not only simplifies your analysis but also enhances the model's performance, making it more accurate and efficient. It's a bit like cleaning a cluttered workspace; once you remove the unnecessary items, you can think more clearly and work more effectively.

Techniques for Feature Selection

Python offers an array of libraries and techniques to aid in feature selection, making it a smooth process. Here, we'll discuss a few popular methods:

Filter Methods: These methods use statistical measures to rank and select features based on their individual relationships with the target variable. Common metrics include correlation coefficients, chi-squared tests, and mutual information. For instance, the SelectKBest function in scikit-learn allows you to select the top K features.

python

```
from sklearn.feature_selection import SelectKBest, chi2

# Select the top 5 features based on chi-squared test
selector = SelectKBest(chi2, k=5)
X_new = selector.fit_transform(X, y)
```

Wrapper Methods: Wrapper methods evaluate different subsets of features by training and testing the model iteratively. Techniques like Recursive Feature Elimination (RFE) can be employed.

python

```
from sklearn.feature_selection import RFE
from sklearn.linear_model import LogisticRegression
```

```
# RFE with a logistic regression model
model = LogisticRegression()
rfe = RFE(model, 5)
fit = rfe.fit(X, y)
```

Embedded Methods: Some machine learning algorithms have built-in feature selection techniques. For example, Lasso and Ridge regression perform feature selection as part of their training process.

python

```
from sklearn.linear_model import Lasso

# Fit a Lasso regression model with feature selection
model = Lasso(alpha=0.01)
model.fit(X, y)
```

Best Practices in Feature Selection

When performing feature selection in healthcare and medical research, it's crucial to keep a few best practices in mind:

Domain Knowledge: Having a good understanding of the healthcare domain is invaluable. Domain experts can provide insights into which features are likely to be relevant.

Regular Updates: Feature selection is not a one-time task. As healthcare data evolves, so do the relevant features. Regularly reevaluate and update your feature selection process.

Benchmarking: Always assess the impact of feature selection on your model's performance. It's possible to remove too much information, so validation is essential.

Visualizations: Data visualization tools can help you understand the relationships between features and the target variable. Tools like Seaborn and Matplotlib can be useful.

Feature selection is a critical step in the data preprocessing pipeline for healthcare and medical research. It ensures that you're working with the most pertinent information, streamlining your analysis and enhancing the performance of your predictive models. In Python, you have a plethora of tools and techniques at your disposal to make this process efficient and effective. Remember, in the world of data, quality often triumphs over quantity. So, choose your features wisely.

Summary and Case Study

In the previous sections of this chapter, we've delved into the crucial realm of data preprocessing in the context of healthcare. We've explored various techniques for preparing healthcare data for analysis, ensuring that it's in the best possible shape to extract meaningful insights. Now, it's time to wrap up this chapter with a concise summary of what we've learned and a compelling case study that puts these data preprocessing techniques into real-world action.

Summary of Data Preprocessing Techniques:

Data preprocessing is the unsung hero of any data analysis endeavor, and in the domain of healthcare, it plays a pivotal role. In this section, we'll recap the key techniques covered in this chapter:

Handling Missing Data: We started by addressing the issue of missing data in healthcare datasets. We discussed strategies such as imputation and removal, ensuring that the integrity of the dataset is maintained.

Outlier Detection and Treatment: Outliers can skew our analysis, so we learned how to identify and handle them effectively, making our results more robust.

Scaling and Normalization: The significance of scaling and normalization in healthcare data became evident. By bringing different features to a common scale, we avoid giving undue importance to certain variables.

Encoding Categorical Data: Healthcare data often contains categorical variables. We explored methods to convert these into a numerical format, making them compatible with data analysis algorithms.

Feature Selection: Not all features are equally relevant in healthcare data. Feature selection techniques allow us to focus on the most informative aspects of our data.

These techniques, when applied diligently, ensure that the data we work with is clean, consistent, and ready for analysis.

Case Study: Enhancing Patient Data for Predictive Modeling

Let's put our knowledge to the test with a practical case study. Imagine you're working for a healthcare provider, and your goal is to develop a predictive model to identify patients at risk of readmission. This model could help allocate resources more efficiently and improve patient care.

Step 1: Handling Missing Data

You start by gathering patient data, but it's far from perfect. Some records have missing values, especially in the vital signs category. Using imputation techniques, you fill in the missing values with statistical estimates, ensuring that no patient is left out of the analysis.

Step 2: Detecting and Treating Outliers

Your data includes outliers in the age and blood pressure fields. Outliers could lead to erroneous predictions, so you apply robust outlier detection methods to identify and correct them.

Step 3: Scaling and Normalization

To ensure that the age and blood pressure features contribute equally to the model, you scale them to a common range, preventing one from dominating the other.

Step 4: Encoding Categorical Data

Patient diagnoses are categorical, and you need to convert them into a numerical format. Using one-hot encoding, you create binary columns for each diagnosis category.

Step 5: Feature Selection

With dozens of potential features, it's vital to select the most relevant ones for your model. You use feature selection techniques like Recursive Feature Elimination (RFE) to identify the critical predictors.

Step 6: Building the Predictive Model

Now that your data is preprocessed, you construct a predictive model using machine learning algorithms. This model takes into account all the preprocessing steps we've discussed, making it a robust tool for predicting readmissions.

Step 7: Model Evaluation and Deployment

After training and fine-tuning your model, you evaluate its performance using metrics like accuracy, precision, and recall. Once satisfied, you deploy it into the healthcare system, where it assists in identifying patients at risk of readmission, ultimately improving patient outcomes.

In this case study, we've seen how the data preprocessing techniques discussed in this chapter are not theoretical concepts but practical tools that can have a significant impact on healthcare outcomes. Clean, well-structured data is the foundation for any successful data analysis or predictive modeling in the medical field.

As you continue your journey through this book, remember that these data preprocessing techniques are just one part of the broader landscape of Python's applications in healthcare. In the chapters to come, you'll explore various facets of Python's role in healthcare research, from data visualization and statistical analysis to machine learning and deep learning in medical imaging. So, let's move forward, armed with the knowledge of how to prepare our data effectively for the exciting adventures that lie ahead.

CHAPTER 6.
STATISTICAL
ANALYSIS

The power of statistics in healthcare research is immeasurable. Statistics are the backbone upon which we build our understanding of medical data, draw critical insights, and make informed decisions. From deciphering patient outcomes to gauging the effectiveness of novel treatments, statistical analysis plays a pivotal role in healthcare's data-driven landscape.

Imagine a world without statistical analysis. We'd be left in the dark, unable to discern whether a new medication is effective or merely a placebo, unable to predict disease trends, or evaluate the efficiency of healthcare systems. Statistics are the guiding light that helps us cut through the complexity of healthcare data.

Statistical analysis equips healthcare professionals with the tools to derive meaningful patterns, identify correlations, and detect outliers within vast datasets. These insights can lead to better patient care, more accurate diagnoses, and cost-effective healthcare solutions.

But it's not just about crunching numbers. Statistical

analysis allows researchers and clinicians to answer pressing questions, such as, "Is a new drug more effective than the existing one?" or "What are the risk factors associated with a particular disease in a given population?" By providing a systematic framework for interpreting data, statistics empower us to make informed decisions that impact individual lives and public health.

Here's where Python, our trusty companion in this journey, steps in. Python offers a rich ecosystem of libraries and tools for statistical analysis. With its -friendly syntax and versatility, it's the ideal language for healthcare professionals and researchers alike.

Let's consider an example to illustrate the importance of statistical analysis in healthcare:

Suppose a pharmaceutical company is developing a new drug to treat a prevalent medical condition. The company conducts clinical trials to test the drug's efficacy, gathering data from hundreds of patients. Without statistical analysis, this mountain of data would be insurmountable, rendering any conclusions unreliable.

However, by applying statistical techniques, researchers can analyze the data to determine whether the new drug yields statistically significant improvements over the current standard of care. They can assess the drug's safety profile and identify potential side effects. Statistical analysis allows them to make data-driven decisions about the drug's viability and, ultimately, its potential to improve patient outcomes.

In Python, you can harness the power of statistical analysis through libraries such as NumPy, SciPy, and StatsModels.

These libraries offer a wide range of statistical tests and methods for hypothesis testing, regression analysis, and much more. Let's look at a simple Python code example that demonstrates hypothesis testing:

```python
import numpy as np
from scipy import stats

# Generate sample data for two groups (e.g., drug and placebo)
group1 = np.array()
group2 = np.array()

# Perform a two-sample t-test to compare means
t_stat, p_value = stats.ttest_ind(group1, group2)

if p_value < 0.05:
    print("There is a statistically significant difference between the two groups.")
else:
    print("No statistically significant difference was found.")
```

In this example, Python is used to conduct a two-sample t-test, a common statistical analysis method. The p-value obtained from the test helps us determine whether there is a significant difference between two groups.

the importance of statistical analysis in healthcare research cannot be overstated. It empowers us to make data-driven decisions, enhance patient care, and advance medical knowledge. With Python as our ally, we have a versatile tool that makes statistical analysis accessible and efficient. So, as we embark on this statistical journey, remember that every data point is a piece of the healthcare puzzle, and statistics help us assemble it into a clearer picture of health and well-being.

Descriptive statistics

Descriptive statistics are like the storytellers of the data world, enabling us to uncover the hidden narratives within healthcare datasets. Whether you're working with patient demographics, treatment outcomes, or any other healthcare-related data, descriptive statistics can help you paint a clear picture.

Measures of Central Tendency:

One of the key aspects of descriptive statistics is measuring central tendency, which includes the mean, median, and mode. The mean is the average value of a dataset, and it provides an overall sense of the data's central position. For example, you could calculate the mean age of patients in a clinical trial.

The median, on the other hand, represents the middle value in a dataset when arranged in ascending order. It's a valuable metric when dealing with datasets that may contain outliers, as it's less affected by extreme values. In healthcare, the median can help identify the typical or middle-ground response to a treatment.

The mode is the value that appears most frequently in a dataset. It's particularly useful when studying categorical data, such as the most common diagnosis within a patient group.

Measures of Variability:

Another critical aspect of descriptive statistics involves measuring the variability of data. This helps us understand how spread out or clustered the data points are. Range, variance, and standard deviation are commonly used to quantify this spread.

The range is simply the difference between the maximum and minimum values in a dataset, offering a quick way to gauge the data's overall variability. For instance, you could calculate the range of blood pressure readings in a patient population.

Variance and standard deviation provide more nuanced measures of data variability. Variance calculates the average of the squared differences from the mean, while the standard deviation is the square root of the variance. These metrics give insights into how data points deviate from the mean, which can be particularly important when assessing the consistency of medical test results.

Visualization Tools:

Descriptive statistics often go hand in hand with data visualization. Histograms, box plots, and frequency distributions help in providing a visual representation of data, making it easier to spot trends and patterns. These tools can be instrumental when analyzing healthcare data, such as patient weight distributions, to identify whether a certain medication affects body weight.

To illustrate, let's consider a hypothetical scenario. Imagine you're analyzing data from a clinical trial testing a new drug's effectiveness. Descriptive statistics can provide you with the average age of the participants (mean), the age at which most participants fall (median), and the most common side effect reported (mode). Moreover, they can help you assess the spread in treatment outcomes (range, variance, and standard deviation), which is crucial in determining the drug's reliability.

Here's a simple Python example to calculate the mean and median ages of trial participants:

python

```python
# Sample list of ages
ages =

# Calculate the mean
mean_age = sum(ages) / len(ages)

# Calculate the median
sorted_ages = sorted(ages)
n = len(sorted_ages)
if n % 2 == 0:
    median_age = (sorted_ages + sorted_ages) / 2
else:
    median_age = sorted_ages

print(f"Mean Age: {mean_age}")
print(f"Median Age: {median_age}")
```

This Python code takes a list of ages, calculates the mean and median, and displays the results. It's just a glimpse into the world of descriptive statistics, which becomes immensely powerful when applied to real healthcare data scenarios.

Normal Distribution (Gaussian Distribution):

The normal distribution, often referred to as the Gaussian distribution, is the bell-shaped curve that many are familiar with. In medical research, it frequently crops up when we're dealing with data such as patients' heights, weights, and blood pressure. The symmetrical nature of the normal distribution makes it an ideal choice when dealing with continuous and symmetric data. This distribution is characterized by two parameters: mean (μ) and standard deviation (σ). In Python, you can use the scipy.stats.norm module to work with the normal distribution.

python

```
import numpy as np
import matplotlib.pyplot as plt
from scipy.stats import norm

# Generate data
data = np.random.normal(0, 1, 1000)

# Plot the probability density function
plt.hist(data, bins=30, density=True, alpha=0.6, color='g')

# Fit a normal distribution to the data
```

```
mu, std = norm.fit(data)
xmin, xmax = plt.xlim()
x = np.linspace(xmin, xmax, 100)
p = norm.pdf(x, mu, std)
plt.plot(x, p, 'k', linewidth=2)
```

Binomial Distribution:

In healthcare research, you might encounter scenarios where you're dealing with binary outcomes, such as the success or failure of a treatment. The binomial distribution models such events, with parameters n (number of trials) and p (probability of success on an individual trial). It's widely used for clinical trials and studies involving binary classification tasks.

Here's a Python example of working with the binomial distribution using the scipy.stats.binom module:

python

```
from scipy.stats import binom

n = 10  # Number of trials
p = 0.3  # Probability of success on each trial

x = np.arange(0, n+1)
pmf = binom.pmf(x, n, p)

plt.vlines(x, 0, pmf, colors='b', lw=5)
plt.title('Binomial Distribution PMF')
```

Poisson Distribution:

The Poisson distribution is commonly used in healthcare to model the occurrence of rare events within a fixed interval. It's applied in epidemiology to predict the number of disease cases, in healthcare logistics for predicting the number of patient arrivals, and more. The Poisson distribution has a single parameter, λ (lambda), which represents the average rate of occurrence.

Here's a Python example for the Poisson distribution:

python

```
from scipy.stats import poisson

lambda_ = 3  # Average rate of occurrence
x = np.arange(0, 11)
pmf = poisson.pmf(x, lambda_)

plt.vlines(x, 0, pmf, colors='r', lw=5)
plt.title('Poisson Distribution PMF')
```

Exponential Distribution:

The exponential distribution is often used to model the time between events in a Poisson process. For instance, it can be used to analyze the time between patient arrivals at a hospital's emergency department. The distribution is characterized by a parameter λ, which represents the rate of events.

Here's a Python example to visualize the exponential distribution:

python

```
from scipy.stats import expon

lambda_ = 0.5  # Rate parameter
x = np.linspace(0, 10, 100)
pdf = expon.pdf(x, scale=1/lambda_)

plt.plot(x, pdf, 'm', lw=2)
plt.title('Exponential Distribution PDF')
```

Understanding these probability distributions is fundamental in healthcare and medical research, as it provides the basis for making informed decisions and predictions. Python's scientific libraries, such as SciPy and NumPy, make it easy to work with these distributions, enabling you to analyze and model medical data effectively. In the subsequent sections of this book, we'll delve deeper into the application of these distributions and other statistical concepts in healthcare research.

Hypothesis Testing

Hypothesis testing is a critical component of healthcare research, allowing us to make informed decisions and draw meaningful conclusions from data. In this section, we'll delve into the principles of hypothesis testing and how it applies to the complex world of medical research.

The Essence of Hypothesis Testing

At its core, hypothesis testing is a statistical method used to determine whether an assumption, or hypothesis, about a population parameter is true. In the context of healthcare research, these hypotheses can be about anything from the effectiveness of a new drug to the impact of a lifestyle change on patient outcomes.

The process begins with two hypotheses:

Null Hypothesis (H0): This is the default assumption that there is no significant effect or difference. It represents the status quo or what we would expect to happen in the absence of any treatment, intervention, or change.

Alternative Hypothesis (H1): This is what we're trying to demonstrate – that there is a significant effect or difference due to a specific intervention, treatment, or condition.

The Steps in Hypothesis Testing

Formulate Hypotheses: Start by defining your null and alternative hypotheses. Be specific about what you're testing and the expected outcome.

H0: The new drug has no significant effect on blood pressure.

H1: The new drug significantly reduces blood pressure.

Collect Data: Gather relevant data, whether it's patient records, clinical trial results, or any other healthcare-related information.

Choose a Significance Level: This is denoted by α (alpha) and represents the probability of making a Type I error (rejecting a true null hypothesis). Common significance levels are 0.05 or 0.01.

Conduct a Test: Based on the data collected, perform a statistical test, such as a t-test or chi-squared test, depending on the nature of your data.

Calculate the Test Statistic: The test statistic helps you quantify the strength of evidence against the null hypothesis. The choice of test determines which formula to use.

Determine the P-Value: The p-value is the probability of observing a test statistic as extreme as the one calculated if the null hypothesis were true. A small p-value (typically less than the chosen significance level) indicates strong evidence against the null hypothesis.

Make a Decision: If the p-value is less than or equal to α, you can reject the null hypothesis in favor of the alternative hypothesis. Otherwise, you fail to reject the null hypothesis.

Python Example

Let's illustrate this with a simple Python example using a fictional dataset of blood pressure measurements before and after administering a new drug.

python

```
import numpy as np
```

```
from scipy import stats

# Sample data
before_drug =
after_drug =

# Perform a paired t-test
t_statistic, p_value = stats.ttest_rel(before_drug, after_drug)

# Set the significance level
alpha = 0.05

# Make a decision
if p_value < alpha:
    print("Reject the null hypothesis: The new drug significantly reduces blood pressure.")
else:
    print("Fail to reject the null hypothesis: There is no significant effect of the new drug on blood pressure.")
```

Hypothesis testing is a powerful tool in healthcare research, allowing us to assess the impact of interventions and treatments. By following a systematic process, researchers can draw meaningful conclusions from data, helping to advance medical knowledge and improve patient care. In the upcoming sections, we will explore further statistical analysis methods and their applications in the field of healthcare research.

Understanding Correlation: Unveiling Hidden Relationships

First, we'll set our sights on correlation analysis. In

the world of healthcare, this technique holds the key to uncovering hidden relationships between variables. It helps us answer questions like, "Does an increase in one variable correlate with an increase or decrease in another?" This kind of insight can be invaluable, whether you're examining the relationship between a patient's age and their cholesterol levels or studying the effect of a specific drug dosage on blood pressure.

We often measure correlation using the Pearson correlation coefficient, symbolized as "r". This coefficient can take values from -1 to 1. A positive "r" value suggests a positive correlation, meaning that as one variable increases, so does the other. Conversely, a negative "r" value indicates a negative correlation, implying that as one variable increases, the other decreases. A value close to zero signifies a weak or no correlation.

Let's illustrate this with a Python example. Suppose we want to explore the correlation between body mass index (BMI) and the risk of heart disease in a given dataset. We can calculate the Pearson correlation coefficient using the numpy library:

python

import numpy as np

Sample data
bmi =
heart_disease_risk =

# Calculate Pearson correlation coefficient
correlation = np.corrcoef(bmi, heart_disease_risk)

print(f"Pearson Correlation Coefficient: {correlation:.2f}")

The output will indicate whether there's a positive or negative correlation between BMI and the risk of heart disease in your dataset.

Unlocking Predictive Insights with Linear Regression

Now, as we grasp the dynamics of correlation, let's segue into the captivating world of linear regression. This technique takes our understanding of relationships between variables to the next level by enabling us to predict one variable based on the other. In healthcare, linear regression is a potent tool for forecasting outcomes, making it indispensable for tasks like predicting patient recovery time or estimating the impact of lifestyle changes on health.

In a linear regression model, we aim to fit a straight line to our data that best represents the relationship between variables. The equation for a simple linear regression model is:

$y = \beta 0 + \beta 1 x y = \beta 0 + \beta 1 x$

Here, "y" represents the dependent variable (the one we want to predict), "x" is the independent variable (the one used for prediction), and $\beta 0 \beta 0$ and $\beta 1 \beta 1$ are the intercept and slope, respectively.

Let's dive into a Python example to grasp this concept better. Suppose we're interested in predicting a patient's blood pressure based on their age. Using the scikit-learn library, we can create a simple linear regression model:

python

```
from sklearn.linear_model import LinearRegression
import numpy as np

# Sample data
age = np.array().reshape(-1, 1)
blood_pressure =

# Create and fit a linear regression model
model = LinearRegression()
model.fit(age, blood_pressure)

# Predict blood pressure for a new age
new_age = np.array([])
predicted_pressure = model.predict(new_age)

print(f"Predicted Blood Pressure: {predicted_pressure:.2f} mm
Hg")
```

In this example, we've trained a linear regression model to predict blood pressure based on age, and we can now use it to make predictions for new data.

As we wrap up this exploration of correlation analysis and linear regression, we've uncovered how these techniques are instrumental in gleaning insights from healthcare data. Whether it's discerning correlations or forecasting outcomes, these tools empower healthcare researchers to make informed decisions and ultimately enhance patient care. In the next section, we'll delve into the fascinating world of Analysis of Variance (ANOVA), adding another layer to our analytical prowess.

Analysis of Variance (ANOVA)

In the vast realm of healthcare research, where the goal is to extract meaningful insights from complex data, statistical methods are the guiding light. Among these methods, Analysis of Variance, or ANOVA, stands out as a powerful tool for examining variations within different groups or treatments. In this section, we will delve into the significance of ANOVA in the context of healthcare research and explore how it can help us draw valuable conclusions from our data.

Understanding Variance and Its Importance:

Before we dive into ANOVA, let's grasp the concept of variance. Variance, in statistics, measures the extent to which data points differ from the mean or average. In healthcare research, variance is often a central focus, as it helps us understand the diversity and deviations in health-related data. For instance, you might be interested in studying the effects of different treatments on patients with a specific medical condition. ANOVA comes into play when you need to determine whether the variations observed among these treatments are statistically significant.

The Anatomy of ANOVA:

Analysis of Variance can be thought of as an extension of the t-test, but with multiple groups. It enables us to compare the means of more than two groups to determine if they are significantly different. In the context of healthcare, this is incredibly useful when we have more than two treatments or interventions to evaluate.

Imagine a scenario in which we're studying the effectiveness of three different drugs in treating a particular disease. Instead of conducting multiple t-tests for each possible pair of drugs, we can use ANOVA to evaluate whether any of the drugs produce significantly different outcomes. In other words, ANOVA helps us answer the question: "Are at least one of these treatments different from the others?"

The Components of ANOVA:

ANOVA breaks down the total variation in the data into two main components: the variation between groups and the variation within groups. The ratio of these variations is used to determine the statistical significance of the differences.

Variation Between Groups: This component measures the differences in means among the various treatment groups. If this variation is large compared to the variation within groups, it suggests that at least one of the treatments is significantly different from the others.

Variation Within Groups: This component quantifies the variability of data points within each group. Smaller variations within groups indicate that the data is more consistent within each treatment group.

Interpreting the ANOVA Results:

When you perform an ANOVA analysis, it will yield a p-value. This p-value indicates whether there are statistically significant differences among the groups. If the p-value is less than a predefined significance level (commonly set at 0.05), you have evidence to suggest that at least one group is different. In such cases, you can proceed with post hoc tests, such as Tukey's HSD, to identify which specific groups are different from each other.

Python Example:

Let's illustrate ANOVA with a Python example. Suppose we have data on the effectiveness of three different exercise regimes on reducing blood pressure in patients. Here, we will use the SciPy library to perform ANOVA.

python

```
import scipy.stats as stats

# Sample data for three exercise regimes
group1 =
group2 =
group3 =

# Performing one-way ANOVA
f_statistic, p_value = stats.f_oneway(group1, group2, group3)

# Checking significance
if p_value < 0.05:
    print("There is a significant difference among the exercise regimes.")
else:
    print("No significant difference found.")
```

In this example, we collected data from three different exercise regimes (group1, group2, and group3) and performed a one-way ANOVA. The result will tell us whether there is a statistically significant difference in their effects on reducing blood pressure.

ANOVA is a fundamental statistical technique that is invaluable in healthcare research. It allows researchers and medical professionals to assess the impact of various treatments, interventions, or factors on patient outcomes. By understanding the variation within and between groups, ANOVA helps identify significant differences and informs evidence-based decision-making in the field of healthcare. This is a powerful tool in your statistical arsenal, and its application in healthcare is wide-ranging and highly relevant.

Non-parametric Statistics

Non-parametric statistics, often referred to as distribution-free statistics, are a vital tool in the healthcare data analyst's toolkit. While the more traditional parametric statistical methods assume a specific data distribution (usually Gaussian), non-parametric statistics make very few assumptions about the underlying data. This flexibility makes them invaluable when dealing with healthcare data, which can often be complex and irregular.

Applicability in Healthcare

In healthcare, we frequently encounter situations where traditional parametric statistics are not suitable. For example, when dealing with ordinal or nominal data, where the assumption of a normal distribution doesn't hold, non-parametric tests come to the rescue. Here are some key scenarios where non-parametric statistics shine:

Ordinal Data Analysis: Non-parametric tests, like the Mann-Whitney U test or the Wilcoxon signed-rank test, are ideal for comparing data that can be ordered but not necessarily assume equal intervals, such as pain scale ratings or patient satisfaction scores.

Categorical Data Analysis: When working with nominal data, like patient blood types or diagnostic categories, non-parametric tests like the Chi-Square test or Fisher's Exact test are crucial for making meaningful comparisons.

Skewed Distributions: In cases where your healthcare data shows significant skewness, non-parametric tests can provide reliable results. This includes scenarios like the distribution of hospital wait times or patient charges.

Small Sample Sizes: Parametric tests often require larger sample sizes to maintain their validity. Non-parametric tests are more robust when dealing with small, limited datasets, which can be common in clinical trials or rare disease studies.

Non-parametric Tests in Python

Now, let's delve into a Python example to illustrate the use of non-parametric statistics. Suppose we have collected data on the recovery times of two different groups of patients, and we want to determine if there's a statistically significant difference between them.

We'll use the Mann-Whitney U test to compare these two groups. Here's a Python code snippet to perform this analysis:

python

```
# Import the required library
from scipy.stats import mannwhitneyu

# Define the data for Group A and Group B
group_a =
group_b =

# Perform the Mann-Whitney U test
statistic, p_value = mannwhitneyu(group_a, group_b)

# Check the results
if p_value < 0.05:  # You can adjust the significance level as needed
    print("There is a statistically significant difference between the groups.")
else:
    print("No statistically significant difference detected.")
```

In this example, we imported the mannwhitneyu function from the scipy.stats library. We then defined our data for Group A and Group B and applied the Mann-Whitney U test. If the p-value is less than our chosen significance level (0.05 in this case), we conclude that there is a statistically significant difference between the two groups.

Non-parametric statistics can empower healthcare professionals to draw robust conclusions from their data, even when it doesn't adhere to the assumptions of parametric tests. These methods are particularly relevant when dealing with patient outcomes, treatment comparisons, and other healthcare-related analyses that involve diverse and sometimes challenging data types.

Remember that while non-parametric tests offer great flexibility, it's crucial to choose the right statistical test for your specific data and research questions. Always ensure that your analysis aligns with the principles of ethical healthcare data research and patient privacy.

Summary and Case Study

As we near the end of our journey through statistical analysis in the realm of healthcare and medical research, it's crucial to reflect on the key concepts we've explored and their real-world applications. This subsection serves a dual purpose: summarizing the essential statistical principles we've covered and presenting a practical case study that illustrates how these principles come together to solve a real problem.

Summarizing Key Statistical Concepts

Throughout this chapter, we've delved into various aspects of statistical analysis and its role in healthcare research. We began by emphasizing the significance of statistics in the healthcare domain, where data-driven decisions can save lives and improve patient outcomes. From there, we journeyed through descriptive statistics, probability distributions, hypothesis testing, correlation and regression, ANOVA, and non-parametric statistics.

In our exploration, we learned how descriptive statistics help us make sense of healthcare data by summarizing it in a meaningful way. Probability distributions became our tools for understanding the likelihood of various medical events. Hypothesis testing allowed us to make informed judgments based on sample data. We also explored the intricacies of correlation and regression, understanding the relationships between different variables in medical datasets.

ANOVA added another layer of complexity, enabling us to compare means across multiple groups, and non-parametric statistics provided alternative methods for analyzing data when assumptions of normality were not met.

In this summary, it's essential to emphasize the practicality of these concepts in healthcare research. From optimizing treatment strategies to identifying risk factors, the statistical tools we've explored are integral to informed decision-making.

Practical Case Study: Improving Patient Outcomes

To bring these concepts to life, let's consider a case study involving a regional healthcare provider aiming to enhance patient outcomes in their cardiac care unit. The objective is to identify factors that influence patient recovery time following heart surgery. Here's how we can apply our statistical knowledge:

Step 1: Data Collection
We gather data on various patient characteristics, such as age, gender, pre-surgery health status, and surgical techniques. Recovery time is recorded as our primary outcome variable.

Step 2: Data Analysis

Using Python, we employ descriptive statistics to gain initial insights into the data. We calculate means, standard deviations, and percentiles for patient age and pre-surgery health status. We visualize the data using box plots and histograms to identify any potential outliers.

Step 3: Hypothesis Testing

We formulate hypotheses: "Age impacts recovery time," and "Surgical technique influences recovery time." We conduct hypothesis tests, such as t-tests and ANOVA, to assess the significance of these factors. Our p-values reveal whether these factors have a substantial impact on recovery time.

Step 4: Regression Analysis

In a multiple linear regression model, we examine the relationships between age, pre-surgery health status, and surgical technique with recovery time. This allows us to quantify the impact of each factor while controlling for others.

Step 5: Recommendations

Based on our analysis, we can provide recommendations to the healthcare provider. For instance, if age is found to significantly affect recovery time, they might consider tailored post-surgery care plans for older patients. Similarly, if surgical technique plays a role, the hospital may explore updated methods.

This case study demonstrates the practical application of the statistical concepts we've covered in this chapter. By analyzing real healthcare data, we can make data-driven recommendations that have the potential to improve patient outcomes and the quality of care provided.

In conclusion, statistical analysis is not just a theoretical endeavor; it's a vital tool in healthcare research that can transform data into actionable insights. By mastering these statistical concepts and their applications, you'll be well-equipped to make a positive impact in the world of healthcare and medical research. The journey doesn't end here; it merely evolves as we move forward into the exciting realm of machine learning for healthcare in the upcoming chapters.

CHAPTER 7. MACHINE LEARNING FOR HEALTHCARE

In the ever-evolving landscape of healthcare, where data is abundant and diverse, the role of machine learning is nothing short of transformative. Welcome to Chapter 7 of our journey through "Python for Healthcare & Medical Research." In this section, we'll delve into the significance of machine learning in healthcare, a field where Python's power truly shines.

Machine learning has become a pivotal player in the healthcare arena, revolutionizing how we approach everything from disease diagnosis to patient care. Python, with its wide array of machine learning libraries and tools, has become the go-to language for healthcare professionals and data scientists alike. So why is machine learning so crucial in the context of healthcare?

The answer lies in the wealth of healthcare data available today. Hospitals, clinics, wearable devices, and even electronic health records (EHRs) generate a staggering amount of data. This data, often referred to as 'big data,' holds invaluable insights that can transform the way we diagnose diseases, personalize treatment plans, and even predict health outcomes.

Machine learning algorithms, which are designed to recognize patterns, can process this vast trove of data, discern meaningful trends, and provide actionable insights. Here are a few key areas where machine learning truly shines in healthcare:

Disease Diagnosis: Machine learning models can analyze medical images, such as X-rays, MRIs, and CT scans, to detect anomalies and diagnose conditions with incredible accuracy. These models can also predict disease risk based on a patient's medical history, genetic information, and lifestyle factors.

Drug Discovery: Machine learning accelerates the drug discovery process by analyzing molecular structures and predicting the effectiveness of potential drugs. This not only saves time but also reduces the cost of developing new medications.

Personalized Medicine: Tailoring treatment plans to individual patients is a dream come true for healthcare. Machine learning can analyze patient data to recommend personalized treatment strategies, medications, and dosages.

Patient Monitoring: Wearable devices and IoT sensors collect real-time patient data, which machine learning algorithms can analyze to provide early warnings for conditions like heart arrhythmias or sudden blood sugar spikes.

Healthcare Operations: Machine learning enhances hospital operations by optimizing resource allocation, predicting patient admissions, and streamlining administrative tasks.

Python's dominance in machine learning stems from its powerful libraries like Scikit-Learn, TensorFlow, and PyTorch. These libraries provide ready-to-use algorithms and tools that enable healthcare professionals to create predictive models without having to reinvent the wheel.

Let's take a brief look at how Python code can be employed in machine learning for healthcare:

python

```
# Example of using Scikit-Learn for a machine learning task
from sklearn.model_selection import train_test_split
from sklearn.ensemble import RandomForestClassifier
from sklearn.metrics import accuracy_score

# Load healthcare data
X, y = load_healthcare_data()

# Split data into training and testing sets
X_train, X_test, y_train, y_test = train_test_split(X, y,
test_size=0.2, random_state=42)

# Create a random forest classifier
clf = RandomForestClassifier(n_estimators=100,
random_state=0)

# Train the model
clf.fit(X_train, y_train)
```

```
# Make predictions on the test set
predictions = clf.predict(X_test)

# Evaluate accuracy
accuracy = accuracy_score(y_test, predictions)
print(f"Accuracy: {accuracy * 100:.2f}%")
```

This Python code demonstrates a typical workflow for training a machine learning model in healthcare. We load our healthcare data, split it into training and testing sets, create a machine learning model (in this case, a Random Forest Classifier), train the model, and evaluate its accuracy.

Scikit-Learn Essentials

In our journey through Python's applications in healthcare and medical research, we've reached a pivotal juncture – the introduction of Scikit-Learn, a powerful library that empowers us to create machine learning models. Scikit-Learn, also known as sklearn, is an essential tool in your Python arsenal when delving into predictive analytics, diagnostic models, and much more within the healthcare domain.

Understanding Scikit-Learn

To put it simply, Scikit-Learn is a comprehensive machine learning library designed to be -friendly and accessible. Its robustness and ease of use make it a valuable resource for both beginners and seasoned data scientists.

Here, we'll embark on a journey to understand the essentials of Scikit-Learn. We'll explore some of the key features, components, and how it can be applied in healthcare contexts.

Setting Up Scikit-Learn

Before we dive into the functionality of Scikit-Learn, we need to ensure that it's correctly installed in your Python environment. If it's not already installed, don't fret; I'll guide you through the process.

python

```
# Install Scikit-Learn using pip
pip install scikit-learn
```

Once installed, we can import the library and start our exploration.

python

```
# Import Scikit-Learn
import sklearn
```

The Anatomy of Scikit-Learn

Scikit-Learn provides a plethora of machine learning tools, including but not limited to:

Supervised Learning Algorithms: These models are trained on labeled data, making predictions based on patterns and relationships within the data. Common supervised learning algorithms include decision trees, support vector machines, and random forests.

Unsupervised Learning Algorithms: In this case, the algorithm explores patterns and structures in data without guidance from labeled outcomes. Clustering and dimensionality reduction are typical tasks within unsupervised learning.

Data Preprocessing Tools: Scikit-Learn offers various tools to prepare your data for analysis. You can handle missing values, scale features, and encode categorical variables.

Model Evaluation: The library includes functions to assess the performance of your machine learning models. Metrics like accuracy, precision, recall, and F1-score come into play when determining how well a model performs in healthcare tasks.

Model Selection: Grid search and cross-validation techniques help you select the best model for your healthcare data.

Building Your First Model

Now, let's roll up our sleeves and build a simple predictive model. Suppose we want to predict the onset of a certain medical condition based on patient data. Here's how you can create a basic decision tree classifier using Scikit-Learn:

python

```
# Import the DecisionTreeClassifier
from sklearn.tree import DecisionTreeClassifier
```

```
# Create an instance of the classifier
clf = DecisionTreeClassifier()

# Train the model using your healthcare dataset
clf.fit(X, y)  # X represents your input features, and y is the
target variable

# Make predictions
predictions = clf.predict(X_new)
```

In this example, DecisionTreeClassifier is just one of the many algorithms Scikit-Learn provides. It's a powerful tool for making predictions based on a decision tree structure.

Scaling Up

As you become more proficient with Scikit-Learn, you can explore more complex algorithms and advanced techniques for model evaluation. Scikit-Learn is renowned for its scalability and versatility, making it suitable for a wide range of healthcare applications.

Remember, the successful application of Scikit-Learn in healthcare doesn't solely rely on knowing how to use the library. It also demands a deep understanding of the healthcare domain, the quality of your data, and the specific questions you aim to answer.

With Scikit-Learn, you're equipped with the tools to build and evaluate machine learning models, advancing your capabilities in healthcare analytics and research. As we progress through this book, you'll further harness the power of

Scikit-Learn in solving real-world healthcare challenges.

Feature Engineering

Feature engineering is the craft of crafting, selecting, and transforming raw data into meaningful features, also known as variables or attributes. These features are the building blocks upon which machine learning models make predictions or classifications. In healthcare data analysis, feature engineering is not just a practice; it's an art, and it's crucial for the success of any data-driven healthcare application.

Why is feature engineering so vital in healthcare, you might ask? The answer lies in the complexity and diversity of healthcare data. In this field, data can take many forms, from patient demographics and lab results to medical imaging and clinical notes. For a machine learning algorithm to effectively learn from this data, it requires well-crafted features that encapsulate relevant information and patterns.

Let's illustrate the significance of feature engineering with a concrete example. Imagine you're developing a predictive model to forecast disease outcomes. Your dataset contains patient records with various attributes, including age, gender, body mass index, and cholesterol levels. These attributes are the raw ingredients of your model. Now, feature engineering steps in to create informative features. You could calculate the patient's age group, categorize the BMI as underweight, normal, overweight, or obese, and determine cholesterol level trends. These derived features provide the model with richer information and help it understand the underlying patterns more effectively.

In Python, libraries like Pandas and NumPy are your trusty allies in the feature engineering journey. You can use Pandas to manipulate and preprocess data efficiently, and NumPy for numerical operations. Let's look at a simple example of feature engineering using Python:

python

```
import pandas as pd

# Sample healthcare dataset
data = {
    'PatientID': ,
    'Age': ,
    'BMI': ,
    'Cholesterol':
}

df = pd.DataFrame(data)

# Create a new feature 'Age Group'
df = pd.cut(df, bins=, labels=)

# Create a new feature 'BMI Category'
df = pd.cut(df, bins=, labels=)

print(df)
```

In this example, we've added two new features, 'Age Group' and 'BMI Category', based on the patient's age and BMI. These engineered features provide a more nuanced understanding of the data, which can significantly impact the model's performance.

Feature engineering isn't a one-size-fits-all process; it requires domain knowledge and creativity to generate the right features for the task at hand. It involves data scaling, normalization, handling missing values, and converting categorical variables into numerical representations, among other techniques. Throughout this book, you'll encounter numerous practical examples of feature engineering tailored to healthcare scenarios, enriching your understanding of this fundamental process.

Remember, the quality of features you engineer can make or break your healthcare predictive model. It's not just about collecting data; it's about transforming it into meaningful insights. So, as you embark on your journey through this chapter and the subsequent ones, keep feature engineering in your toolkit and wield it wisely. It's the secret sauce that can turn your healthcare data into actionable knowledge.

Supervised Learning

Supervised learning, a pivotal domain of machine learning that plays a crucial role in the analysis of medical data. Supervised learning is the keystone upon which predictive models are built. This technique enables us to train our algorithms by providing them with labeled data, allowing them to learn and make predictions based on the patterns and relationships within that data. It's akin to a teacher guiding a student, providing answers to specific problems, until the student can solve similar problems on their own.

In the context of healthcare and medical research, supervised learning is akin to having an expert physician guide us in understanding patient data, making diagnoses, and even predicting future health outcomes. This powerful tool has a myriad of applications, such as disease diagnosis, patient risk assessment, and treatment recommendation systems. But how does it work, and how can we apply it in the context of Python programming?

The crux of supervised learning lies in the training of predictive models. These models are like digital physicians, equipped with the ability to analyze medical data and make informed decisions. To illustrate the concept, let's delve into a simple example using Python, and demonstrate how to build a basic supervised learning model.

python

```
# Import the necessary libraries
from sklearn.model_selection import train_test_split
from sklearn.tree import DecisionTreeClassifier
from sklearn.metrics import accuracy_score

# Assume we have a dataset with patient information,
including age, BMI, and blood pressure.
# Our task is to predict whether a patient has hypertension
based on this data.

# Load the dataset (your data source may vary)
data = load_patient_data()
```

```
# Split the data into features (X) and target (y)
X = data]
y = data

# Split the dataset into a training set and a testing set
X_train, X_test, y_train, y_test = train_test_split(X, y,
test_size=0.2, random_state=42)

# Create a decision tree classifier
model = DecisionTreeClassifier()

# Train the model on the training data
model.fit(X_train, y_train)

# Make predictions on the testing data
y_pred = model.predict(X_test)

# Calculate the accuracy of the model
accuracy = accuracy_score(y_test, y_pred)

print(f"Model Accuracy: {accuracy}")
```

In this example, we've used Python's scikit-learn library to create a basic decision tree classifier. We loaded a hypothetical patient dataset, split it into features (age, BMI, and blood pressure) and the target variable (hypertension), and then divided the data into training and testing sets. The model was trained on the training data and subsequently used to make predictions on the testing data. The accuracy of the model was evaluated using the accuracy_score function.

This is just a glimpse of what supervised learning can achieve in healthcare and medical research. With more complex algorithms and larger datasets, the possibilities are endless. From predicting diseases to assisting in medical image analysis, supervised learning is a potent tool for extracting valuable insights from healthcare data.

Furthermore, advancements in Python libraries and frameworks, as well as the integration of new healthcare-related datasets, are continually expanding the horizons of what we can accomplish. The future of healthcare and medical research is intertwined with the promise of machine learning, and mastering supervised learning is a pivotal step on that path.

Unsupervised Learning

In the vast realm of healthcare and medical research, data often comes in abundance. We're inundated with information, from patient records to diagnostic images and everything in between. Making sense of this wealth of data can be a daunting task, and that's where unsupervised learning steps in as our trusty guide. So, let's embark on a journey to explore the world of unsupervised learning and understand its applications in the context of healthcare.

Unsupervised learning, as the name suggests, stands in contrast to supervised learning, where we don the hats of teachers guiding the algorithm with labeled data. In unsupervised learning, there are no predefined answers or labels to guide our model. Instead, it ventures into the uncharted territory of raw data to discover patterns, hidden structures, and relationships on its own.

Clustering: A Fundamental Approach

One of the primary applications of unsupervised learning in healthcare is clustering. Clustering algorithms are akin to expert cartographers, grouping similar data points together on the map of your dataset. These algorithms detect patterns and categorize data into clusters based on inherent similarities. The applications are vast, from patient segmentation to disease classification.

Imagine you have a dataset containing medical records of thousands of patients, each described by various attributes like age, gender, medical history, and more. Unsupervised learning algorithms can sift through this data and group patients with similar characteristics into distinct clusters. This can lead to valuable insights for personalized treatment plans and predicting disease risk.

Dimensionality Reduction: Simplifying Complexity

Healthcare data is notorious for its high dimensionality, with a multitude of variables to consider. Unsupervised learning offers dimensionality reduction techniques that enable us to simplify complex data without losing crucial information. Principal Component Analysis (PCA) is a stellar example. It identifies the most significant components within your data, allowing you to focus on the essentials.

For instance, think of medical imaging data that includes thousands of pixels in high-resolution scans. By employing PCA, you can reduce this vast pixel data into a handful of essential components, retaining the key information while significantly simplifying subsequent analyses.

Anomaly Detection: Finding Needles in Haystacks

In the healthcare landscape, finding anomalies can be a matter of life and death. Unsupervised learning methods are our trusty anomaly detectors. They sift through extensive datasets, identifying data points that deviate significantly from the norm. This is invaluable in spotting rare diseases, unusual patient responses to treatments, or even fraud detection in health insurance claims.

Natural Language Processing (NLP): Unlocking the Power of Text

In the world of healthcare, a substantial portion of data exists in unstructured text format—clinical notes, research papers, patient records, and more. Unsupervised learning, when coupled with NLP, can help make sense of this textual wealth. It extracts meaning from the unstructured, turning it into structured knowledge. Topic modeling, for example, can unveil the themes within medical literature, aiding in research and decision-making.

Case Study: Patient Segmentation

Let's dive into a practical example. Consider a hospital that wants to segment its patients for more personalized care. The dataset contains various attributes: age, medical history, diagnoses, and response to treatments. Unsupervised learning comes to the rescue. It clusters patients into distinct groups, each with its own unique characteristics.

For instance, one cluster might consist of elderly patients with chronic conditions, while another could be young adults with sports injuries. These segments enable healthcare providers to tailor treatment plans and interventions according to each group's specific needs.

Python in Action

Now, let's shift our focus to practical Python examples. Python offers a myriad of libraries and tools for unsupervised learning. One such powerful library is Scikit-Learn. Here's a brief snippet to demonstrate how you can use K-Means clustering to segment patients:

python

```
from sklearn.cluster import KMeans

# Assuming 'data' is your patient dataset
kmeans = KMeans(n_clusters=3)  # Specify the number of clusters
kmeans.fit(data)

# The cluster labels for each patient
patient_clusters = kmeans.labels_
```

In this example, we've used K-Means to group patients into three clusters. The resulting 'patient_clusters' array provides the cluster assignment for each patient. These clusters can then guide personalized care.

Evaluating Model Performance

Before selecting the best model, it's essential to evaluate their performance. In this context, performance refers to how well a model can make predictions or classifications based on the provided data. Common metrics for evaluating model performance include accuracy, precision, recall, F1 score, and the area under the receiver operating characteristic curve (AUC-ROC).

For instance, in a healthcare setting, you might be interested in classifying medical images as either "normal" or "abnormal." In such a case, accuracy measures the overall correctness of predictions, while precision and recall assess the model's ability to correctly identify abnormal cases without many false alarms. AUC-ROC provides insights into the model's ability to distinguish between the two classes.

Let's take a look at a Python example for calculating these performance metrics:

python

```
from sklearn.metrics import accuracy_score, precision_score, recall_score, f1_score, roc_auc_score

# Assuming you have true labels and predicted labels
true_labels =
predicted_labels =

accuracy = accuracy_score(true_labels, predicted_labels)
precision = precision_score(true_labels, predicted_labels)
recall = recall_score(true_labels, predicted_labels)
```

```
f1 = f1_score(true_labels, predicted_labels)
roc_auc = roc_auc_score(true_labels, predicted_labels)

print(f"Accuracy: {accuracy}")
print(f"Precision: {precision}")
print(f"Recall: {recall}")
print(f"F1 Score: {f1}")
print(f"AUC-ROC Score: {roc_auc}")
```

By calculating these metrics, you can make informed decisions about your model's performance.

Cross-Validation

Model evaluation also involves techniques like cross-validation, which assesses how well your model will generalize to unseen data. Cross-validation splits your dataset into multiple subsets, training the model on one and testing on the others, and then repeating this process multiple times. It provides a more robust estimate of a model's performance.

Hyperparameter Tuning

Choosing the right hyperparameters for your machine learning models can significantly impact their performance. Grid search and randomized search are two common methods for hyperparameter tuning. These techniques involve systematically testing various combinations of hyperparameters to find the best set for your specific problem.

Here's a Python example using scikit-learn for hyperparameter tuning:

python

```
from sklearn.model_selection import GridSearchCV
from sklearn.ensemble import RandomForestClassifier

# Define the hyperparameters and their potential values
param_grid = {
    'n_estimators': ,
    'max_depth':
}

# Create the model
model = RandomForestClassifier()

# Use grid search to find the best hyperparameters
grid_search = GridSearchCV(model, param_grid, cv=5)
grid_search.fit(X, y)

best_params = grid_search.best_params_
print(f"Best Hyperparameters: {best_params}")
```

Model Selection

Once you've evaluated multiple models with various metrics, it's time to select the best one for your healthcare data. The choice depends on your specific research goals and the nature of the data. For instance, a random forest model might work well for tabular clinical data, while a convolutional neural network (CNN) is suitable for medical image analysis.

The process of model evaluation and selection is iterative and might involve going back to the data preprocessing and feature engineering steps. It's important to remember that the "best" model is the one that aligns most closely with your research objectives and the characteristics of your healthcare dataset.

The selection of the right machine learning model is a pivotal step in the journey of using Python for healthcare and medical research. By carefully evaluating model performance, implementing cross-validation, tuning hyperparameters, and considering the specific needs of your project, you can choose the model that will ultimately yield the most accurate and reliable results. The next subsection, 7.7b, will delve into advanced topics in healthcare ML, further expanding your knowledge in this critical field.

Advanced Topics in Healthcare ML

Machine learning in healthcare is more than just prediction and classification. It's about harnessing the full potential of data to drive innovation, optimize treatments, and save lives. As you continue your journey into the world of healthcare machine learning, you'll encounter advanced topics that push the boundaries of what's possible. Let's explore some of these captivating areas:

Ensemble Learning: In the dynamic landscape of healthcare, combining the predictions of multiple models can lead to more accurate and robust results. Ensemble techniques like Random Forests, Gradient Boosting, and AdaBoost become essential tools for improving diagnostic accuracy, predicting patient outcomes, and optimizing resource allocation in hospitals.

Imbalanced Data Handling: Healthcare datasets often suffer from class imbalances. When you're dealing with rare diseases or anomalies, traditional machine learning algorithms can struggle. Advanced methods like SMOTE (Synthetic Minority Over-sampling Technique) and ADASYN (Adaptive Synthetic Sampling) come to the rescue by rebalancing datasets, ensuring your models are sensitive to critical minority classes.

Time Series Analysis: Many healthcare datasets involve a temporal component. Whether it's patient records, monitoring data, or clinical trials, understanding how data evolves over time is crucial. Time series analysis and forecasting techniques enable healthcare professionals to anticipate disease progression, patient deterioration, and even healthcare resource demand.

Interpretable Machine Learning: The "black-box" nature of some machine learning models can be a concern in healthcare, where decisions can have life-altering consequences. Interpretable machine learning techniques, such as LIME (Local Interpretable Model-Agnostic Explanations) and SHAP (SHapley Additive exPlanations), help reveal the reasoning behind model predictions, increasing trust and aiding clinical decision-making.

Transfer Learning in Healthcare: Leveraging pre-trained models for healthcare applications can significantly speed up the development of AI-driven solutions. Transfer learning allows you to adapt models trained on large, general datasets to healthcare tasks, reducing the need for massive labeled datasets and expediting innovation.

Explainable AI in Healthcare: Understanding why a model

makes a specific prediction is paramount in healthcare. Explainable AI, through methods like decision trees, rule-based systems, and feature importance analysis, provides a transparent view of the decision-making process, making it easier for healthcare professionals to trust AI recommendations.

Advanced Application Example: Predicting Disease Outcomes

Let's consider a practical application. Imagine you're working on a project to predict patient outcomes in a hospital's intensive care unit (ICU). This is a complex task that requires an advanced machine learning approach.

You have access to a vast dataset comprising patient demographics, vital signs, lab results, and treatment histories. By employing ensemble learning, you can combine the strengths of various models to provide more accurate predictions. Additionally, interpretable machine learning techniques help healthcare professionals understand why a particular patient is at higher risk, ensuring they can make well-informed decisions.

Moreover, time series analysis allows you to create dynamic predictions. You can monitor a patient's condition over time and provide updated forecasts, giving clinicians a valuable tool for proactive care.

These advanced topics are the frontier of machine learning in healthcare. As you continue your journey through this chapter, you'll gain the expertise to tackle these challenges, opening the door to groundbreaking innovations in the field of healthcare.

Remember, healthcare is a realm where every prediction, every diagnosis, and every decision matters profoundly. Advanced machine learning techniques are not just tools; they are the key to shaping the future of healthcare and saving lives.

Supervised Learning and Unsupervised Learning

We started our exploration by distinguishing between supervised and unsupervised learning. In supervised learning, we employ labeled data to train models for tasks like classification and regression. These models can predict patient outcomes, diagnose diseases, and optimize treatment plans. Unsupervised learning, on the other hand, is invaluable for clustering and dimensionality reduction, helping to uncover hidden patterns and relationships within healthcare data.

Feature Engineering and Model Evaluation

Machine learning success hinges on feature engineering, where you select and preprocess the right attributes from your dataset. This process ensures that your model can uncover meaningful insights. Remember that a well-engineered feature set can dramatically enhance your model's performance. But choosing the appropriate evaluation metrics is equally crucial for assessing how well your model is performing. Metrics like accuracy, precision, recall, and F1-score are vital in the healthcare domain.

Advanced Topics in Healthcare ML

We also explored advanced topics in healthcare machine learning, such as imbalanced data handling, ensembling methods, and handling electronic health records (EHR) data.

These advanced techniques are essential for addressing the complex challenges unique to healthcare datasets. They allow us to create robust models that can make a real impact on patient care and medical research.

Ethical Considerations and Data Privacy

Throughout your journey into machine learning for healthcare, always keep ethical considerations and data privacy at the forefront of your decision-making process. Healthcare data is sensitive and subject to stringent regulations. Therefore, it's crucial to understand how to handle data responsibly, maintain patient privacy, and adhere to regulations like HIPAA.

Chapter Summary

In summary, Chapter 7 has equipped you with the essential knowledge and skills to embark on your machine learning journey in healthcare. You've learned about supervised and unsupervised learning, feature engineering, model evaluation, and advanced topics in healthcare machine learning. Moreover, you've gained insights into the ethical considerations and privacy concerns associated with healthcare data.

As you move forward, continue to explore the vast landscape of machine learning in healthcare. Stay updated on the latest developments in the field, as it is constantly evolving. Real-world applications of machine learning in healthcare, such as predictive disease modeling, personalized treatment recommendations, and image analysis, are transforming the industry. Your journey in this exciting field is just beginning, and you are well-prepared to contribute to the advancement of healthcare through the power of Python and machine learning.

With your newfound knowledge and skills, you have the potential to make a significant impact on healthcare research, patient outcomes, and the overall well-being of society. Keep learning, experimenting, and applying your expertise to drive positive change in the world of healthcare. Thank you for joining us on this enlightening journey through the intersection of Python and healthcare. Your contribution to this vital field is greatly anticipated.

CHAPTER 8. DEEP LEARNING FOR MEDICAL IMAGING

In the realm of medical image analysis, we delve into the cutting-edge world of deep learning. This is a frontier of artificial intelligence that has revolutionized the way we interpret and derive insights from medical images, such as X-rays, MRIs, CT scans, and even histopathological slides. Deep learning has made it possible for computers to not only 'see' images but to 'understand' them on a level previously reserved for human experts.

Deep learning is a subset of machine learning, and it's inspired by the human brain's structure and function. It employs artificial neural networks to recognize complex patterns and representations in data, especially images. In the context of healthcare, deep learning has found myriad applications, with medical image analysis being one of the most prominent and impactful.

So, why is deep learning so pivotal in medical image analysis? The answer lies in its ability to unearth intricate patterns, anomalies, and details that might escape the human eye. This technology can assist healthcare professionals in making faster, more accurate diagnoses and treatment decisions. Let's delve deeper into why deep learning has become a game-changer in the field.

Uncovering Subtle Patterns:

Medical images often contain subtle and nuanced patterns that can be indicative of various conditions. These patterns may not be readily discernible by the naked eye or through traditional image processing techniques. Deep learning models, particularly Convolutional Neural Networks (CNNs), have shown remarkable proficiency in detecting these subtle patterns. For instance, in the early detection of diseases like cancer, deep learning models can identify minuscule irregularities in medical images, offering the possibility of early intervention and improved patient outcomes.

Automation and Efficiency:

In the past, analyzing medical images was a time-consuming and labor-intensive process, often requiring human experts to scrutinize each image thoroughly. Deep learning automates this process, significantly reducing the time it takes to analyze images. This not only increases the efficiency of healthcare but also ensures that more patients can receive timely diagnoses and treatment.

Large-Scale Data Analysis:

Deep learning thrives on large volumes of data. In the context of medical image analysis, it can process and derive insights from extensive datasets containing thousands, or even millions, of images. The more data the model is trained on, the more accurate and robust it becomes. This makes it ideal for the vast repositories of medical images that healthcare institutions accumulate over time.

Personalized Medicine:

Deep learning enables the practice of personalized medicine. By considering an individual's unique medical history and genetic makeup, deep learning algorithms can tailor diagnoses and treatment plans to specific patients. This precision can lead to more effective and efficient healthcare, reducing the likelihood of adverse reactions and improving patient satisfaction.

The Road Ahead:

The future of deep learning in healthcare is incredibly promising. As technology advances, so too will the capabilities of deep learning models. We can expect even more accurate diagnoses, faster image processing, and the discovery of new, previously unidentified patterns within medical images. Additionally, deep learning is likely to play a crucial role in other areas of healthcare, such as drug discovery and predictive analytics.

Now that we've explored the significance of deep learning in medical image analysis, you might wonder how these complex neural networks function. To provide you with a glimpse into the inner workings of deep learning, let's delve into a simplified example. Below is a Python code snippet that demonstrates a basic convolutional neural network designed for image classification:

python

```
import tensorflow as tf
```

```
from tensorflow.keras import layers, models

# Create a simple convolutional neural network
model = models.Sequential()

model.add(layers.Conv2D(32, (3, 3), activation='relu',
input_shape=(64, 64, 3)))
model.add(layers.MaxPooling2D((2, 2)))
model.add(layers.Conv2D(64, (3, 3), activation='relu'))
model.add(layers.MaxPooling2D((2, 2)))
model.add(layers.Conv2D(64, (3, 3), activation='relu'))

model.add(layers.Flatten())
model.add(layers.Dense(64, activation='relu'))
model.add(layers.Dense(10, activation='softmax'))

# Compile the model
model.compile(optimizer='adam',
        loss='sparse_categorical_crossentropy',
        metrics=)

# Now you can train the model with your medical image
dataset
```

This is just a simplified example, but it illustrates the core principles of a convolutional neural network used in deep learning for image analysis. Deep learning is an expansive field with numerous libraries and tools at your disposal. As you embark on your journey into the world of deep learning, you'll explore more intricate models and gain a deeper understanding of their capabilities in the context of medical image analysis.

Understanding Convolutional Neural Networks (CNNs)

At the core of the matter, a Convolutional Neural Network is a specialized deep learning model tailored for image-related tasks. CNNs have revolutionized the way we approach medical imaging, offering unparalleled capabilities in tasks such as image classification, segmentation, and even object detection.

Let's break down how CNNs work. Imagine you have a vast collection of medical images, each holding crucial information. Traditional neural networks may struggle to analyze these images due to their sheer complexity and size. This is where CNNs step in as the heroes of the story.

The Convolution Process

CNNs are inspired by the human visual system. They 'learn' to recognize patterns, features, and structures within images through a process called convolution. This process involves a series of convolutional layers, each with specialized filters that scan the input image.

As the filters sweep across the image, they detect distinctive features, like edges, shapes, and textures. These features are gradually combined, allowing the network to learn more complex patterns. In the context of medical imaging, CNNs can identify tumors, anomalies, or any other critical information hidden within the images.

Pooling and Fully Connected Layers

But the journey doesn't stop there. After the convolutional layers, CNNs often include pooling layers. These layers reduce the spatial dimensions of the data, making it computationally more manageable while retaining essential information. Following the pooling layers, fully connected layers are employed to make sense of the features extracted from the images.

Applications in Medical Imaging

CNNs are the backbone of many advanced medical imaging applications. They can assist in diagnosing diseases, precisely locating anomalies, and even tracking the progression of illnesses. For example, they can analyze X-rays, MRIs, or CT scans to identify tumors, fractures, or abnormalities.

In the realm of pathology, CNNs are used to examine microscopic slides, assisting pathologists in identifying cellular structures and anomalies that might escape the human eye. This significantly speeds up the diagnostic process and enhances its accuracy.

Moreover, CNNs find applications in monitoring the progress of treatments. By comparing medical images taken at different times, these networks can detect subtle changes that could signify improvement or deterioration in a patient's condition.

Real-World Implementation

To truly appreciate the impact of CNNs in healthcare, consider an example. Imagine a CNN analyzing a series of MRI scans from a patient with a brain tumor. The network can not only identify the tumor's location and size but also track its growth over time. This real-time analysis is invaluable for doctors and can influence treatment decisions, ultimately improving patient care.

In the field of radiology, CNNs have become invaluable partners to radiologists. By rapidly screening through massive datasets, they help identify potential issues, allowing human experts to focus their attention on critical cases.

Python Programming Example

Here's a simplified Python code snippet to give you a glimpse of how to create a basic CNN using popular deep learning libraries such as TensorFlow and Keras:

python

```python
import tensorflow as tf
from tensorflow import keras

# Create a sequential model
model = keras.Sequential()

# Add convolutional layers
model.add(keras.layers.Conv2D(32, (3, 3), activation='relu',
input_shape=(128, 128, 3)))
model.add(keras.layers.MaxPooling2D((2, 2)))

# Add fully connected layers
model.add(keras.layers.Flatten())
model.add(keras.layers.Dense(64, activation='relu'))
```

```
model.add(keras.layers.Dense(10, activation='softmax'))
```

This example represents a simplified CNN for image classification. In a real-world medical imaging scenario, the model architecture would be more complex, tailored to the specific task.

Convolutional Neural Networks are the backbone of modern medical imaging, empowering healthcare professionals to make accurate and timely diagnoses. Their ability to 'see' beyond what the human eye can perceive has transformed the field of healthcare. As we progress through this chapter, we'll dive deeper into the practical aspects of building and training CNNs for medical image analysis, bringing the power of deep learning closer to your grasp.

Image Preprocessing for Medical Images

In medical imaging, the quality of the images plays a pivotal role in diagnosis and analysis. However, raw medical images often come with imperfections, noise, and variations that can complicate the interpretation process. To mitigate these challenges and prepare images for subsequent analysis, a crucial step in any medical imaging pipeline is image preprocessing.

Why Preprocessing Matters

Before diving into the specific techniques for image preprocessing, let's understand why it matters. Medical images, whether from X-rays, MRIs, CT scans, or other modalities, are often acquired under less-than-ideal conditions. Factors like patient movement, sensor limitations, and the presence of artifacts can lead to suboptimal images.

Therefore, preprocessing is essential for the following reasons:

Enhancing Image Quality: Preprocessing techniques aim to improve the quality of medical images by reducing noise, correcting artifacts, and enhancing details. This leads to better diagnostic accuracy and more informative data for analysis.

Standardization: Standardizing the images ensures that they have consistent brightness, contrast, and size. This is crucial when comparing images across different patients or time points.

Feature Extraction: Many image analysis tasks rely on extracting specific features or regions of interest. Preprocessing helps in segmenting and extracting these features effectively.

Reducing Computational Load: In some cases, medical images can be massive in size. Preprocessing techniques can help reduce the computational burden by resizing or compressing images while preserving essential information.

Now, let's delve into the key preprocessing techniques used in the medical imaging domain.

Noise Reduction

Noise can significantly degrade the quality of medical images. Techniques like Gaussian smoothing, median filtering, or wavelet denoising are applied to reduce noise. Here's a Python example using the OpenCV library to perform Gaussian smoothing:

python

```python
import cv2
import numpy as np

# Load the medical image
image = cv2.imread('medical_image.png')

# Apply Gaussian smoothing
smoothed_image = cv2.GaussianBlur(image, (5, 5), 0)

# Display the smoothed image
cv2.imshow('Smoothed Image', smoothed_image)
cv2.waitKey(0)
cv2.destroyAllWindows()
```

Contrast Enhancement

Enhancing the contrast of medical images can reveal important details. Techniques like histogram equalization or contrast stretching are commonly used. Here's a Python example for histogram equalization using OpenCV:

python

```python
# Load the medical image
image = cv2.imread('medical_image.png', 0)

# Apply histogram equalization
equalized_image = cv2.equalizeHist(image)
```

```
# Display the equalized image
cv2.imshow('Equalized Image', equalized_image)
cv2.waitKey(0)
cv2.destroyAllWindows()
```

Normalization and Scaling

Standardizing pixel values to a specific range, such as , can be crucial. This step ensures that images are consistent in terms of intensity levels. Here's a Python example for min-max scaling:

python

```
# Load the medical image
image = cv2.imread('medical_image.png', 0)

# Min-max scaling
scaled_image = cv2.normalize(image, None, 0, 255,
cv2.NORM_MINMAX)

# Display the scaled image
cv2.imshow('Scaled Image', scaled_image)
cv2.waitKey(0)
cv2.destroyAllWindows()
```

Artifact Correction

Artifacts in medical images can distort the diagnostic information. Depending on the type of artifact, specific techniques are applied. For instance, geometric correction algorithms can rectify distortions caused by imaging sensors.

Resizing and Cropping

Resizing medical images to a consistent resolution or cropping to focus on regions of interest are common preprocessing steps. Python's OpenCV library is handy for these operations.

python

```
# Resize the medical image to a specific width and height
resized_image = cv2.resize(image, (new_width, new_height))
```

Image preprocessing for medical images is a vast field, and the choice of techniques depends on the specific imaging modality and analysis goals. These techniques aim to ensure that the images are in the best possible condition for subsequent tasks, whether it's disease detection, image segmentation, or feature extraction.

By applying these preprocessing techniques, the medical imaging community can harness the power of deep learning, computer vision, and other advanced technologies to make more accurate diagnoses and contribute to improved patient care.

Building the Foundation

To commence our venture into CNNs, it's essential to first understand their architecture. CNNs are composed of multiple layers, primarily including convolutional layers, pooling layers, and fully connected layers. These layers are designed to capture, and process features of the input images progressively.

Convolutional Layers: These layers are the workhorses of CNNs. They consist of numerous filters that slide over the input image to detect various patterns and features. Convolutional layers can capture intricate details, such as edges, shapes, and textures.

Pooling Layers: After convolution, pooling layers reduce the spatial dimensions of the data. They help in simplifying the information while retaining the essential features. This step reduces computational load and combats overfitting.

Fully Connected Layers: The final layers of a CNN are fully connected, transforming the learned features into predictions. These layers make decisions based on the data's processed features.

Training the Network:

Once we've established our network's architecture, the next step is training. Training a CNN involves presenting it with a labeled dataset of medical images, allowing the network to learn patterns and features. Here's a breakdown of this process:

Data Preparation: A crucial aspect of training is data preparation. You need a substantial dataset of medical images, meticulously labeled with corresponding diagnoses or annotations. This dataset forms the basis for training and evaluation.

Loss Function: To gauge how well the CNN is performing, a

loss function is defined. This function measures the disparity between the network's predictions and the actual labels. The objective is to minimize this loss.

Optimization: An optimization algorithm, like Stochastic Gradient Descent (SGD) or Adam, is employed to adjust the network's internal parameters (weights and biases). These adjustments are made iteratively to minimize the loss.

Backpropagation: As the network processes data and calculates loss, it simultaneously performs backpropagation. This is the process of adjusting the model's parameters in reverse order, optimizing them for better accuracy.

Validation and Testing: Throughout training, it's essential to validate the model's performance using a separate dataset not seen during training. This helps assess the model's generalization capabilities. Testing is done to evaluate the fully trained model on new, unseen data.

Fine-Tuning: Depending on the results from validation and testing, the model may undergo fine-tuning. This involves making adjustments to the architecture, optimizing hyperparameters, or acquiring more data if necessary.

Python Code Examples:

To grasp the technical aspects better, let's illustrate these concepts with Python code examples. Below is a simplified Python code snippet that demonstrates the creation and training of a basic CNN using the TensorFlow and Keras libraries:

python

```python
import tensorflow as tf
from tensorflow import keras

# Define the CNN model
model = keras.Sequential()

# Compile the model
model.compile(optimizer='adam',
        loss='sparse_categorical_crossentropy',
        metrics=)

# Train the model
model.fit(train_images,     train_labels,     epochs=10,
validation_data=(val_images, val_labels))
```

This code defines a simple CNN architecture, compiles it with necessary settings, and trains it on medical images.

Building and training CNNs for medical image analysis is a complex yet rewarding process. It empowers us to extract valuable insights from images, aiding in diagnoses and treatments. As you explore this field further, remember that practice, patience, and continuous learning are your allies on this exciting journey.

The Essence of Transfer Learning

Transfer learning operates on the notion that knowledge acquired from one task can be used to improve learning in another. In the domain of medical imaging, this means we can take neural networks pre-trained on a vast dataset of generic images, such as ImageNet, and fine-tune them for medical image analysis tasks. The advantage is apparent: we begin with a model that already possesses a substantial understanding of features and patterns, and then we adapt it for a specific medical task.

To accomplish this, Python provides a plethora of libraries, including TensorFlow and PyTorch, that offer pre-trained models and tools to facilitate transfer learning. Let's explore the steps involved in the process.

Steps in Transfer Learning with Python

Select a Pre-trained Model: Begin by choosing a pre-trained model that aligns with your medical image analysis task. Common choices include VGG, ResNet, or Inception. You can easily load these models using Python libraries like TensorFlow or PyTorch.

Modify the Top Layers: Since the top layers of the pre-trained model are specialized for the original task (e.g., object recognition), you need to adapt them for your specific medical image analysis task. In Python, you can do this by replacing or adding new layers to the model.

Data Preparation: Prepare your medical image dataset. This includes labeling the data and augmenting it if necessary. Python libraries like OpenCV and Pillow come in handy for image preprocessing.

Training: Utilize the modified pre-trained model and fine-tune it on your medical dataset. Python's deep learning frameworks provide the necessary tools for this step, making it relatively straightforward.

Evaluation: Once the model is trained, assess its

performance using metrics like accuracy, precision, and recall. Python libraries like scikit-learn can assist in evaluating the model's effectiveness.

Fine-tuning and Iteration: Depending on the evaluation results, you may need to fine-tune the model further. Python's flexibility allows for quick adjustments and iterations.

Applications in Healthcare

The applications of transfer learning in healthcare are extensive. For instance, consider the task of diagnosing skin cancer from dermoscopic images. By employing a pre-trained model, initially created for general image recognition, and fine-tuning it with a dataset of skin images, you can create a powerful diagnostic tool.

Another application lies in the interpretation of X-rays and MRIs. Transfer learning can help in identifying anomalies and diseases within these medical images, aiding radiologists in their diagnoses.

In the field of medical imaging, rapid progress is being made through transfer learning, thanks to Python's accessibility and the wealth of pre-trained models readily available. This approach not only saves time but also ensures the development of highly accurate models, contributing significantly to improved patient care.

The power of Python lies in its robust ecosystem of libraries, which simplifies complex tasks like transfer learning. Whether you're a seasoned data scientist or a newcomer to the field, Python offers the tools you need to harness the capabilities of pre-trained models and apply them to the intricate world of medical image analysis. With dedication and the right resources at your disposal, you can make a substantial impact in healthcare through the application of transfer learning.

Object Detection and Segmentation

In the realm of medical imaging, the ability to accurately detect and segment objects of interest is nothing short of revolutionary. This process involves identifying specific structures within images, often essential for diagnosis, treatment planning, and research. In this section, we'll delve into the fascinating world of object detection and segmentation in medical images, exploring both the critical need for these techniques and the methods to achieve them using Python.

The Significance of Object Detection and Segmentation

Imagine a medical scenario where a physician needs to locate and measure the size of tumors in an MRI scan or identify blood vessels in an angiogram. These tasks are daunting without the aid of technology. This is where object detection and segmentation come into play.

Object Detection: This technique is the first step. It involves identifying the presence of specific objects within an image. In medical imaging, these objects can be tumors, organs, or anomalies. Python's powerful libraries and tools, particularly deep learning frameworks, allow us to build models that can detect these objects with remarkable accuracy.

Segmentation: Once we've identified the objects, the next challenge is to accurately outline and separate them from the rest of the image. This is what segmentation accomplishes. It helps in precisely defining the boundaries of the object of interest. Python offers several libraries and algorithms for image segmentation, making it an indispensable tool in healthcare image analysis.

Python's Role in Object Detection and Segmentation

Python, being a versatile programming language, provides an array of libraries and frameworks that make object detection and segmentation tasks more accessible. Two of the most prominent ones are TensorFlow and PyTorch. These deep learning frameworks offer pre-trained models that can be fine-tuned for specific medical imaging tasks.

TensorFlow: TensorFlow, developed by Google, is known for its flexibility and support for deep learning models. Its ecosystem includes high-level APIs like Keras, making it -friendly for those who are just getting started with deep learning. In the context of medical image analysis, TensorFlow's object detection API can be leveraged for identifying regions of interest within images. It provides pre-trained models that can be fine-tuned for specific medical applications.

PyTorch: Developed by Facebook's AI Research lab, PyTorch is lauded for its dynamic computation graph and strong support in the research community. PyTorch's pre-trained models and easy-to-follow tutorials facilitate the implementation of object detection and segmentation tasks for medical images. Its - friendly nature makes it an excellent choice for researchers and practitioners in the healthcare domain.

An Example of Object Detection and Segmentation in Python

To illustrate the concept, let's consider a scenario: the detection and segmentation of lung nodules in chest X-ray images. We'll use Python, along with the PyTorch library, to build a simple model. First, we need to prepare our data, which consists of a dataset of chest X-ray images with labeled lung nodules.

python

```python
# Import necessary libraries
import torch
import torch.nn as nn
import torch.optim as optim
from torchvision import transforms, models

# Define a custom deep learning model for object detection
class LungNoduleDetector(nn.Module):
    def __init__(self):
        super(LungNoduleDetector, self).__init__()
        # Define the layers of your model here

    def forward(self, x):
        # Implement the forward pass here
        pass

# Load the dataset, define data loaders, and choose a loss function and optimizer

# Training loop to fine-tune the model for lung nodule detection
```

Implement the segmentation part to outline the detected nodules

Visualize and evaluate the results

This example represents a simplified workflow for object detection and segmentation. In practice, the model architecture, data preparation, and optimization require more in-depth consideration, but it serves as a starting point for your journey into this exciting field.

Case Studies in Medical Image Analysis

Case Study 1: Automated Tumor Detection

Imagine a scenario where early detection of tumors becomes not just a possibility but a reality. Deep learning models, particularly Convolutional Neural Networks (CNNs), have made significant strides in automating tumor detection through medical imaging.

In this case study, we explore the development of a CNN-based model for the early detection of breast cancer using mammograms. The process involves preprocessing the medical images, training the model, and evaluating its performance. By the end of this case study, readers will gain a comprehensive understanding of how deep learning can assist radiologists and oncologists in identifying potential malignancies swiftly and accurately.

python

```python
# Python code example
import tensorflow as tf
from tensorflow.keras.preprocessing.image import ImageDataGenerator

# Data preprocessing and augmentation
train_datagen = ImageDataGenerator(
    rescale=1./255,
    shear_range=0.2,
    zoom_range=0.2,
    horizontal_flip=True
)

# Building a Convolutional Neural Network
model = tf.keras.Sequential()

# Model compilation and training
model.compile(loss='binary_crossentropy', optimizer='adam', metrics=)
```

Case Study 2: Neuroimaging for Disease Diagnosis

Neuroimaging, which includes techniques like MRI and fMRI, plays a pivotal role in the diagnosis of neurological disorders. Deep learning models offer the capability to automate the interpretation of these complex images.

In this case study, we explore how Python, particularly the TensorFlow library, is used to create a model that can analyze brain scans and detect abnormalities. We'll delve into the intricacies of building and training a Convolutional Neural Network that can distinguish between healthy brain scans and those indicative of conditions such as Alzheimer's disease. The potential here is not just in enhancing diagnostic accuracy but also in significantly reducing the time required for diagnosis.

python

```python
# Python code example
import tensorflow as tf
from tensorflow.keras.layers import Conv2D, MaxPooling2D, Flatten, Dense
from tensorflow.keras.models import Sequential

# Building a Convolutional Neural Network
model = Sequential()

# Model compilation and training
model.compile(loss='binary_crossentropy', optimizer='adam', metrics=)
```

These two case studies provide a glimpse into the immense potential of deep learning in the field of medical image analysis. Python's extensive libraries and frameworks, combined with the power of deep neural networks, have the capacity to revolutionize how we detect and diagnose diseases, ultimately leading to better patient outcomes.

In the coming chapters, we'll continue to explore practical applications of Python in healthcare, including natural language processing, ethical considerations, and emerging technologies. The journey into the world of Python for healthcare and medical research is a dynamic and ever-evolving one, offering exciting opportunities to those willing to embark on it.

]

]

In the previous chapter, we embarked on an exciting journey into the realm of deep learning for medical imaging. We delved into the intricacies of Convolutional Neural Networks (CNNs), explored image preprocessing techniques, and learned how to build and train CNNs for the analysis of medical images. With each step, we got closer to unraveling the immense potential of Python in the field of healthcare.

As we wrap up this chapter, let's take a moment to reflect on the key concepts and applications we've covered. Deep learning is not just a buzzword; it's a transformative force in the world of medical imaging.

We began by discussing the pivotal role of deep learning in medical image analysis. This technology has revolutionized the way medical professionals interpret and diagnose various conditions, from detecting tumors in radiological images to segmenting anatomical structures with high precision.

Our journey continued with an exploration of Convolutional Neural Networks (CNNs), which are the workhorses behind many breakthroughs in medical imaging. You learned how

CNNs are specifically designed to process visual data, making them exceptionally adept at tasks like classifying diseases from X-ray images or identifying abnormalities in MRI scans.

To ensure the data fed into these networks is optimal, we examined image preprocessing techniques. This step is crucial to enhance image quality, remove noise, and standardize the data for the best possible model performance. Remember, clean data is the foundation of accurate deep learning.

Building and training CNNs is an art form in itself. We discussed the architecture of CNNs, how layers interact, and the training process. The model's ability to generalize and make predictions depends on the quality and quantity of your training data, and the hyperparameters you fine-tune.

Transfer learning opened the door to leveraging pre-trained models and adapting them for specific medical imaging tasks. By doing so, you can save time and computational resources while achieving remarkable results. This approach is a testament to the efficiency of Python in healthcare.

Object detection and segmentation represent the pinnacle of image analysis. We explored how deep learning can not only identify objects of interest in medical images but also delineate their boundaries with incredible precision. These techniques are pivotal in tasks like localizing tumors or anatomical structures.

To illustrate the real-world impact of deep learning in healthcare, we delved into practical case studies. These examples showcased how Python and deep learning are applied in scenarios such as disease detection, medical image diagnosis, and more. The possibilities are vast, and the results are awe-inspiring.

As we conclude this chapter, remember that deep learning is more than just a set of algorithms. It's a beacon of hope for the healthcare industry. With Python as your tool, you can contribute to the advancement of medical science, improve patient outcomes, and make a real difference in the world.

In the upcoming chapters, we will continue our exploration of Python's applications in healthcare. But for now, take a moment to appreciate the incredible journey you've undertaken. The world of deep learning is vast, and you're well on your way to mastering it.

So, as we move forward, armed with knowledge and enthusiasm, let's continue to explore the incredible possibilities that Python offers in the field of healthcare. There are more discoveries to be made, and you're in the driver's seat, ready to make a positive impact.

CHAPTER 9.
NATURAL LANGUAGE PROCESSING (NLP)

The role of technology in healthcare continues to evolve and expand. Python, with its versatility and adaptability, has found a profound place in this field. One of the most intriguing applications of Python in healthcare is Natural Language Processing, or NLP.

Why is NLP such a game-changer in the realm of healthcare, and why should you, as a healthcare professional or researcher, be excited about its potential? Well, let's embark on a journey to uncover the significance of NLP in healthcare.

The Power of Language

Imagine a world where patient records, medical research papers, and clinical notes could be instantly analyzed, categorized, and interpreted by a computer system. This is the promise of NLP. In a domain where information is abundant but often buried within the confines of unstructured text, NLP emerges as a beacon of hope.

Healthcare is replete with textual data, from electronic health records (EHRs) to clinical trial reports and medical literature.

The ability to extract meaningful insights from this wealth of information is crucial for medical professionals, researchers, and healthcare institutions. This is precisely where NLP steps in.

Deciphering the Narrative

Natural Language Processing is the technology that empowers computers to understand, interpret, and generate human language. In the context of healthcare, this means that machines can read and make sense of the textual data generated every day in clinical settings, laboratories, and medical journals.

NLP techniques enable the extraction of critical information from clinical notes, allowing healthcare providers to quickly identify patient histories, treatment plans, and adverse events. Researchers can efficiently analyze vast amounts of scientific literature to discover trends and insights that might otherwise remain hidden.

Clinical Decision Support

One of the most significant contributions of NLP to healthcare is in clinical decision support. By processing the natural language in EHRs, NLP systems can alert healthcare providers to potential drug interactions, recommend treatments based on the latest medical research, and even assist in the diagnosis of diseases by identifying relevant symptoms and medical histories.

Imagine a scenario where a physician, while examining a patient's electronic health record, receives real-time suggestions and warnings regarding potential complications or alternative treatment options. NLP makes this scenario not just possible but increasingly practical.

Efficiency and Precision

In a time-critical environment like healthcare, the speed and precision of information retrieval can make all the difference. NLP algorithms are designed to swiftly sift through mountains of textual data and pinpoint the exact details that matter. This efficiency translates to quicker decision-making, reduced administrative burden, and ultimately, improved patient care.

A Glimpse into the Future

As we progress through this book, you'll delve deeper into the world of NLP in healthcare. We'll explore text preprocessing techniques, sentiment analysis, and the development of healthcare chatbots. We'll see how NLP can be applied to clinical text data, unleashing its potential for clinical research and patient care.

With Python as our toolkit, we're ready to unlock the doors to a new era of healthcare where data-driven insights are not confined to structured databases but extend to the vast realms of human language. Together, we'll navigate the fascinating landscape of NLP in healthcare, equipping you with the knowledge and skills to harness its transformative power.

Text Preprocessing

Before diving into the intricacies of healthcare text data analysis, it's essential to prepare the textual information for meaningful insights. Text preprocessing is the initial step in this journey. Its significance lies in enhancing the quality of text data, making it more manageable and facilitating the application of natural language processing (NLP) techniques.

One of the primary challenges in working with healthcare text data is its inherent noise. Text data often contains irrelevant information, special characters, and formatting issues. To extract valuable insights and patterns, we need to clean and transform the data. Here's a step-by-step guide on how to do that:

1. Text Lowercasing

Begin by converting all text to lowercase. This standardizes the text and ensures that words are not treated differently due to their capitalization. For example, 'Heart' and 'heart' should be recognized as the same word.

2. Tokenization

Tokenization involves splitting the text into individual words or tokens. It's a critical step to analyze the structure of sentences and understand the relationships between words. In Python, the Natural Language Toolkit (NLTK) library provides efficient tokenization functions.

3. Removing Stop Words

Stop words are common words like 'the,' 'and,' 'in,' which don't contribute much to the meaning of a sentence. Eliminating stop words can reduce noise in the data and help focus on relevant content.

4. Removing Special Characters and Punctuation

Healthcare text often contains special characters, punctuation marks, and symbols that may not be necessary for analysis. Removing them streamlines the text data.

5. Lemmatization and Stemming

Lemmatization and stemming are techniques to reduce words to their base or root forms. For instance, 'running' becomes 'run,' and 'happily' becomes 'happy.' This process aids in identifying the core meaning of words.

6. Handling Synonyms and Abbreviations

In healthcare, synonyms and medical abbreviations are prevalent. Text preprocessing should include mechanisms to map these variations to a common representation. For example, 'cardiac arrest' and 'heart attack' should be recognized as synonymous.

7. Spell Checking and Correction

Accurate text data analysis hinges on proper spelling. Implementing spell-checking mechanisms can enhance the quality of the text, reducing ambiguities caused by typos.

8. Handling Negations and Context

Negations can reverse the meaning of phrases. For example, 'not effective' is different from 'effective.' Text preprocessing should consider the context in which negations appear to avoid misinterpretations.

Python Code Examples:

python

```
# Example of text preprocessing in Python using NLTK
import nltk
from nltk.corpus import stopwords
from nltk.tokenize import word_tokenize
from nltk.stem import WordNetLemmatizer

# Sample text data
text = "The patient didn't have any complications after the surgery. It was highly successful."

# Step 1: Convert to lowercase
text = text.lower()

# Step 2: Tokenization
tokens = word_tokenize(text)

# Step 3: Removing stop words
stop_words = set(stopwords.words('english'))
filtered_tokens =

# Step 4: Removing punctuation and special characters
filtered_tokens =

# Step 5: Lemmatization
```

```
lemmatizer = WordNetLemmatizer()
lemmatized_tokens =

print(lemmatized_tokens)
```

These are just some of the essential techniques for text preprocessing in healthcare data analysis. By implementing these strategies, you can ensure that your text data is ready for more advanced NLP tasks, such as sentiment analysis, text classification, and named entity recognition.

Text preprocessing sets the stage for unlocking the valuable insights hidden within healthcare text data. Whether you're working on clinical notes, patient reviews, or medical research papers, a well-preprocessed text can be the key to making informed decisions and advancing healthcare research. So, dive into the world of text preprocessing and harness the power of healthcare text data for the betterment of medical science.

Sentiment Analysis: Decoding Emotions in Healthcare Text

Healthcare records, patient feedback, and even medical publications contain a wealth of textual data. Sentiment analysis involves the use of natural language processing (NLP) techniques to determine the emotions and sentiments expressed in this data. By understanding the emotional tone of the text, healthcare providers and researchers can gauge patient satisfaction, identify areas of improvement, and even predict outbreaks or public health concerns.

Consider a scenario where patient feedback is collected through surveys or online reviews. Sentiment analysis can automatically analyze this feedback, sorting it into categories like positive, negative, or neutral. For instance, a positive sentiment might indicate patient satisfaction with the care received, while negative sentiment could reveal areas of concern or dissatisfaction.

Here's a Python example that demonstrates sentiment analysis using the popular NLP library, NLTK:

python

```
import nltk
from nltk.sentiment.vader import import
SentimentIntensityAnalyzer

# Sample healthcare feedback
feedback = "The healthcare services provided were excellent. I am very satisfied."

# Initialize the sentiment analyzer
analyzer = SentimentIntensityAnalyzer()

# Analyze sentiment
sentiment_scores = analyzer.polarity_scores(feedback)

# Determine sentiment category
if sentiment_scores >= 0.05:
    sentiment_category = "positive"
elif sentiment_scores <= -0.05:
    sentiment_category = "negative"
else:
```

```python
sentiment_category = "neutral"
```

```python
print(f"Sentiment: {sentiment_category}")
```

By examining the compound score from the sentiment analysis, you can classify the sentiment as positive, negative, or neutral, aiding in a quick overview of patient feedback.

Text Classification: Organizing Healthcare Text

Text classification, another crucial component of NLP, involves categorizing healthcare text into predefined classes. In the healthcare domain, this could include categorizing medical reports into different specialties, tagging clinical notes with relevant conditions, or classifying research papers based on their focus areas.

Python, with libraries like scikit-learn, offers robust tools for text classification. Here's a simplified example of classifying clinical notes:

python

```python
from sklearn.feature_extraction.text import TfidfVectorizer
from sklearn.naive_bayes import MultinomialNB
from sklearn.pipeline import make_pipeline
```

```python
# Sample clinical notes and their categories
clinical_notes =
```

```python
categories =
```

```
# Create a text classification model
model = make_pipeline(TfidfVectorizer(), MultinomialNB())

# Train the model
model.fit(clinical_notes, categories)

# Predict the category of a new clinical note
new_note = "The patient's heart shows irregularities."
predicted_category = model.predict()

print(f"Predicted Category: {predicted_category}")
```

Text classification helps streamline information retrieval and organization, enabling healthcare professionals and researchers to efficiently access the data they need.

By diving into sentiment analysis and text classification in healthcare, you're embarking on a journey to unlock the potential of textual data in this critical field. These NLP techniques provide valuable insights, streamline operations, and, most importantly, enhance patient care. As you delve deeper into Python and its NLP capabilities, you'll find the tools you need to make a significant impact in the healthcare domain.

Named Entity Recognition (NER)

Named Entity Recognition, or NER, stands as a crucial pillar in the realm of healthcare data analysis. In this section, we delve into the significance of NER and its indispensable role in identifying healthcare entities.

Healthcare data often comes in the form of unstructured text, from clinical notes and medical reports to research articles and patient records. Extracting valuable information from this wealth of data can be a daunting task. That's where Named Entity Recognition steps in as the unsung hero of healthcare informatics.

Imagine poring through thousands of patient records or research papers, searching for mentions of medical conditions, medications, or patient names. This manual effort is not only time-consuming but prone to errors. NER, powered by Python, automates this process with remarkable precision and efficiency.

Let's break it down further. Named Entity Recognition involves identifying and categorizing entities within the text, such as names of diseases, medications, healthcare facilities, and even dates. Python offers a wide array of libraries and tools for NER, making it accessible and practical for healthcare professionals, data analysts, and researchers.

For example, the Natural Language Toolkit (NLTK) and spaCy are Python libraries that boast powerful NER capabilities. These libraries can swiftly scan through texts and recognize entities like "Hypertension," "Aspirin," "Mayo Clinic," or "January 15, 2023." With this information, you can derive invaluable insights for various healthcare applications, including disease trend analysis, adverse drug reaction monitoring, or patient history extraction.

Here's a simplified Python example demonstrating NER using spaCy:

python

```python
import spacy

# Load the spaCy model for NER
nlp = spacy.load("en_core_web_sm")

# Sample healthcare text
healthcare_text = "The patient was diagnosed with Type 2 Diabetes on March 12, 2022, and prescribed Metformin."

# Process the text with spaCy
doc = nlp(healthcare_text)

# Extract and categorize entities
for ent in doc.ents:
    print(f"Entity: {ent.text}, Category: {ent.label_}")
```

In this code snippet, we first load the spaCy model for NER, and then we process a sample healthcare text. The output will provide you with recognized entities and their corresponding categories. It's a small glimpse of the powerful NER capabilities that Python brings to the table.

NER is indispensable for healthcare professionals and researchers, as it streamlines data extraction, enables comprehensive analysis, and aids in making informed decisions. It's a shining example of how Python empowers the healthcare field with efficient tools and techniques.

Building Healthcare Chatbots

Before we jump into the technical aspects, it's essential to grasp the pivotal role healthcare chatbots play in the industry. These intelligent conversational agents are engineered to serve several key functions:

Appointment Scheduling: Healthcare chatbots can efficiently handle appointment bookings, cancellations, and rescheduling, saving time for both patients and healthcare providers. They work around the clock, ensuring that no time slot goes unfilled.

Symptom Assessment: They can assist s in assessing their symptoms, providing preliminary insights into potential health issues. Chatbots use advanced algorithms to ask relevant questions and offer preliminary advice.

Medication Reminders: For patients with chronic conditions, staying on top of medication schedules is crucial. Healthcare chatbots can send timely reminders, ensuring that patients adhere to their prescribed treatments.

Health Information: Chatbots can be a valuable source of health information. They can answer questions about common medical conditions, explain treatment options, and provide general health tips.

Emergency Assistance: In critical situations, chatbots can offer guidance on immediate actions to take before professional medical help arrives.

Developing Healthcare Chatbots with NLP and Python

Now, let's explore how these chatbots are created using

Natural Language Processing, a branch of artificial intelligence focused on enabling machines to understand and generate human language.

1. Data Collection: Building an effective healthcare chatbot begins with gathering a diverse dataset of healthcare-related conversations and questions. This dataset is used to train the chatbot's language model.

2. NLP Libraries: Python offers a rich ecosystem of NLP libraries, with the Natural Language Toolkit (NLTK) and spaCy being two prominent choices. These libraries provide essential tools for text processing, tokenization, and linguistic analysis.

3. Language Model: The heart of any chatbot is its language model. Pre-trained models like OpenAI's GPT (Generative Pre-trained Transformer) can be fine-tuned on healthcare-specific data to make the chatbot contextually aware.

4. Intent Recognition: Understanding the intent behind a 's query is crucial. Python's libraries, combined with machine learning techniques, can help in intent recognition. For instance, a asking, "What are the symptoms of COVID-19?" should trigger the symptom assessment function.

5. Dialog Flow: Designing a logical and empathetic dialog flow is vital. Python's frameworks like Django and Flask can be used to create a web-based interface for the chatbot, allowing it to interact with s.

6. Entity Recognition: Identifying and extracting healthcare entities from queries, such as medications, symptoms, or conditions, is another NLP task. Python libraries and machine learning models are applied for this purpose.

7. HIPAA Compliance: Healthcare chatbots must adhere to strict privacy regulations like HIPAA in the United States. Python's robust security libraries help ensure that data remains confidential and secure.

8. Testing and Validation: Thorough testing is essential to iron out any kinks in the chatbot's responses. Python's testing frameworks, such as pytest, are used to automate the testing process.

9. Continuous Learning: Healthcare is an ever-evolving field. Python's versatility allows chatbots to be continuously updated with the latest medical knowledge and guidelines.

10. Experience: A good healthcare chatbot provides an excellent experience. This is achieved through a combination of NLP, Python, and thoughtful design that anticipates needs and provides clear, empathetic responses.

In conclusion, healthcare chatbots represent a remarkable intersection of technology and patient care. By leveraging Python's NLP capabilities, you can embark on a journey to create chatbots that enhance the efficiency of healthcare delivery, provide valuable information, and improve patient outcomes. The synergy between NLP and Python is powering a healthcare revolution, making information and support more accessible to everyone.

So, whether you're a developer, a healthcare professional, or simply curious about the future of healthcare, Python's capabilities in the realm of NLP offer a gateway to explore this exciting frontier.

Clinical Text Analytics

Clinical text data contains a treasure trove of unstructured information. It comprises physician notes, patient histories, radiology reports, and more. However, making sense of this unstructured data requires sophisticated text analytics techniques.

Python, as a versatile programming language, offers a multitude of tools and libraries that can be applied to clinical text analytics. Let's dive into some key methods and tools that researchers and healthcare professionals can leverage to unlock the secrets hidden within clinical text data.

Natural Language Processing (NLP): The Foundation of Clinical Text Analytics

At the core of clinical text analytics lies Natural Language Processing (NLP), a subfield of artificial intelligence that focuses on the interaction between computers and human language. Python's NLP libraries, such as NLTK (Natural Language Toolkit), spaCy, and TextBlob, provide powerful capabilities for processing and analyzing text data.

For instance, NLP techniques can be used to perform:

Named Entity Recognition (NER): Identifying and categorizing entities such as medical conditions, drug names, and patient names within text.

Sentiment Analysis: Assessing the emotional tone of clinical notes, which can be valuable for understanding patient sentiments or healthcare provider opinions.

Text Classification: Categorizing clinical text into predefined categories, which can be used for tasks like routing medical records or classifying radiology reports.

Python Example: Named Entity Recognition

python

```
import spacy

# Load the English NLP model
nlp = spacy.load("en_core_web_sm")

# Sample clinical text
clinical_text = "The patient was prescribed 100mg of aspirin for hypertension."

# Process the text with spaCy
doc = nlp(clinical_text)

# Extract named entities
named_entities =

print(named_entities)
```

The code above demonstrates how to use spaCy to perform Named Entity Recognition on clinical text data. It identifies "aspirin" as a medication and "hypertension" as a medical condition.

Challenges and Solutions

Clinical text analytics is not without its challenges. Clinical notes can be riddled with misspellings, acronyms, and medical jargon. However, Python's libraries allow for the development of custom solutions to address these challenges. Leverage techniques like text normalization, stemming, and lemmatization to enhance the accuracy of clinical text analysis.

Real-world Applications

The applications of clinical text analytics are far-reaching. For instance, it can aid in the automated extraction of relevant patient information from electronic health records, assist in clinical decision support, and contribute to the detection of adverse drug events.

Moreover, research and epidemiological studies can benefit from the analysis of large-scale clinical text data, as it provides valuable insights into disease trends and treatment effectiveness.

Summary and Case Study

In this final section of the Natural Language Processing (NLP) chapter, we will tie together all the essential concepts we've explored in the realm of healthcare text analysis using Python. NLP is an exciting field with wide-ranging applications in healthcare, from understanding patient sentiments in medical records to building intelligent chatbots that can provide support and answer medical queries. We've traversed through the intricacies of text preprocessing, sentiment analysis, named entity recognition, and clinical text analytics. Now, it's time to summarize and consolidate our knowledge.

Summary of Key NLP Concepts:

NLP, in the context of healthcare, is all about extracting meaningful information from textual data. Here's a brief overview of what we've learned:

Introduction to NLP: We started by understanding the significance of NLP in healthcare, emphasizing the abundance of unstructured clinical text data.

Text Preprocessing: Text data can be messy and unstructured, and preprocessing is the first step. We explored techniques like tokenization, stemming, and stop-word removal to clean and prepare the text.

Sentiment Analysis and Text Classification: Sentiment analysis allows us to gauge the emotional tone within text, which is crucial for understanding patient sentiments or feedback. Text classification, on the other hand, helps categorize texts into predefined classes, aiding in tasks like disease classification.

Named Entity Recognition (NER): NER enables the identification of specific entities within text, such as diseases, drugs, or clinical procedures. This is particularly useful in extracting structured information from clinical notes.

Building Healthcare Chatbots: We delved into the development of healthcare chatbots, which can assist patients, answer their questions, and provide information on various medical topics. Python's NLP capabilities make this possible.

Clinical Text Analytics: We showcased how text analytics methods can be applied to clinical text data, helping researchers and healthcare professionals extract valuable insights from a vast amount of textual information.

Case Study: Enhancing Healthcare Patient Support with an NLP Chatbot

Let's bring our understanding to life with a case study. Imagine a healthcare provider that wants to improve patient support by offering a 24/7 virtual assistant. They decide to build a chatbot that can answer patient queries, provide information about common medical conditions, and even schedule appointments. The goal is to enhance the overall patient experience and alleviate the burden on human staff.

Python, with its powerful NLP libraries, is the perfect tool for this task. Here's how the process unfolds:

Data Collection: The healthcare provider collects historical patient queries and responses. This data forms the basis for training the chatbot.

Text Preprocessing: The collected text data is preprocessed. This includes tasks like removing stop words, stemming, and tokenization to ensure the text is ready for analysis.

Training the Chatbot: Using machine learning techniques, the chatbot is trained on the preprocessed data. It learns to understand patient queries and provide appropriate responses.

Sentiment Analysis: The chatbot is equipped with sentiment

analysis capabilities. This allows it to gauge the emotional tone of patient queries and respond with empathy and understanding.

Named Entity Recognition: NER is used to identify medical entities in the text. This helps the chatbot provide accurate information about diseases, treatments, and medications.

Continuous Learning: The chatbot is not static. It continually learns from new patient interactions, improving its responses and accuracy over time.

Integration: The chatbot is integrated into the healthcare provider's website and mobile app, making it easily accessible to patients.

As a result of implementing this chatbot, the healthcare provider experiences a significant improvement in patient support. Patients can get quick answers to their questions, schedule appointments without delay, and feel more connected with the provider. This case study exemplifies the practical application of NLP in healthcare, enhancing the patient experience through intelligent virtual assistants.

In conclusion, Natural Language Processing is a pivotal field in the healthcare industry, bridging the gap between the wealth of unstructured textual data and actionable insights. By understanding the core NLP concepts and their real-world applications, you're well-equipped to navigate the ever-evolving landscape of healthcare informatics. Whether it's sentiment analysis, entity recognition, or building chatbots, Python is your ally in harnessing the power of healthcare text data for the benefit of patients and medical professionals alike.

CHAPTER 10.
HEALTHCARE DATA
ETHICS AND PRIVACY

A crucial aspect in healthcare data that demands our attention is the ethical considerations that govern its usage. In this section, we delve into the core principles that guide the responsible handling of healthcare data, emphasizing the significance of ethical choices in healthcare informatics.

In today's digital era, healthcare data isn't just numbers and text; it's a representation of individuals' health, privacy, and even their lives. Understanding the ethical implications of using this data is paramount.

The Heart of Data Ethics

Ethical considerations in healthcare data usage encompass a myriad of aspects, but a central theme is ensuring the well-being and privacy of patients. At its core, data ethics involves the responsible collection, storage, processing, and sharing of healthcare data, with a profound respect for individuals' rights and interests.

Data ethics in healthcare extends beyond legal compliance. While regulations like HIPAA (Health Insurance Portability and Accountability Act) provide a legal framework for safeguarding patient data, true data ethics goes above and beyond the law. It requires us to question not just "Is this legal?" but also "Is this the right thing to do?"

Privacy Matters

One of the most prominent ethical considerations in healthcare data is patient privacy. Every piece of healthcare data, from medical records to lab results, contains sensitive information about individuals. Respecting their privacy is paramount.

Consider a scenario where a researcher has access to a large dataset of patient records. While the data may be de-identified, meaning it doesn't contain names or direct identifiers, there's still a risk of re-identification. Ethical data handling requires the researcher to employ the highest standards of privacy protection, ensuring that no individual can be traced back through the data.

Transparency and Informed Consent

Another vital aspect of data ethics is transparency. Individuals should know how their data is being used and have the right to grant or deny consent. In healthcare, this means that patients should be informed about how their data will be utilized, and their consent should be obtained before any data is shared or used for research.

Researchers and data scientists must be transparent about their intentions and methodologies. Openly sharing the purpose of data usage, the steps taken to protect privacy, and the potential benefits of research builds trust and aligns with ethical standards.

Minimizing Harm and Maximizing Good

Data ethics also involve the principles of minimizing harm and maximizing good. When working with healthcare data, researchers should aim to minimize any potential harm that may befall individuals due to data breaches or unethical use. Simultaneously, they should seek to maximize the good that can come from their research, such as improved treatments, diagnoses, or public health policies.

For example, if a study using healthcare data identifies a severe health risk in a specific population, ethical considerations dictate that this information should be communicated to the concerned individuals and healthcare providers. This approach minimizes harm by allowing early intervention and maximizes good by potentially saving lives.

Ethical Dilemmas in Data Sharing

Data ethics in healthcare can often lead to ethical dilemmas. For instance, striking a balance between privacy and public health interests during a pandemic can be a significant challenge. While sharing data for tracking and controlling the spread of a contagious disease is vital, it must be done in a way that safeguards individuals' privacy.

The Role of Data Stewards

Data ethics isn't just a matter for researchers and data scientists; it involves all stakeholders who handle healthcare data, including healthcare providers, institutions, and policymakers. They play a vital role in defining and enforcing ethical standards.

In essence, the ethical considerations in healthcare data usage revolve around a profound respect for individuals' rights, privacy, and well-being. Data ethics isn't a set of rules to follow; it's a mindset that underpins every action in the healthcare data domain.

In subsequent sections of this book, we will explore various strategies and techniques for maintaining data ethics in healthcare. These include anonymization and de-identification methods, privacy regulations, and security measures to prevent data breaches. We will equip you with the knowledge and tools to ensure that ethical considerations are at the forefront of your healthcare data endeavors.

Remember, ethical data usage isn't just a requirement; it's an essential part of advancing healthcare and medical research responsibly.

Privacy Regulations in Healthcare

Privacy in healthcare is not merely a legal requirement but a fundamental ethical concern. In this section, we delve into the critical aspect of privacy regulations, with a particular focus on the Health Insurance Portability and Accountability Act (HIPAA), which plays a pivotal role in safeguarding patient information.

Understanding the HIPAA:

Privacy in healthcare is paramount, as it involves the most sensitive and personal data – an individual's health records. To ensure that this data is handled with the utmost care and confidentiality, the United States enacted the HIPAA in

1996. HIPAA is a multifaceted legislation that encompasses both Privacy and Security Rules. It sets the standards for the protection of patients' medical records and other personal health information.

HIPAA Privacy Rule, in a nutshell, controls who has access to a patient's healthcare records. Covered entities, such as healthcare providers, health plans, and healthcare clearinghouses, must comply with this rule. They are required to provide patients with a Notice of Privacy Practices explaining how their health information is used, and they must obtain written consent from patients before sharing their data.

HIPAA Security Rule, on the other hand, focuses on the protection of electronic patient health information (ePHI). It sets standards for the secure transmission and storage of electronic health records. This rule impacts not only healthcare providers but also their business associates, such as data storage and IT companies.

Compliance with HIPAA:

For healthcare organizations and professionals, compliance with HIPAA is not optional. It is a legal obligation. Failure to comply with HIPAA can result in severe penalties, both in terms of fines and reputation. As a result, healthcare entities invest heavily in data security measures, staff training, and audits to ensure they adhere to HIPAA standards.

Let's look at a Python example illustrating data encryption to comply with HIPAA Security Rule:

python

```python
import cryptography
from cryptography.fernet import Fernet

# Generate a key for encryption
key = Fernet.generate_key()
cipher_suite = Fernet(key)

# Data to be encrypted
sensitive_data = "Patient: John Doe, DOB: 01/15/1980, Diagnosis: Hypertension"

# Encrypt the data
encrypted_data                                    =
cipher_suite.encrypt(sensitive_data.encode())

# Decrypt the data (only authorized personnel should have access to the key)
decrypted_data                                    =
cipher_suite.decrypt(encrypted_data).decode()

print("Original Data: ", sensitive_data)
print("Encrypted Data: ", encrypted_data)
print("Decrypted Data: ", decrypted_data)
```

In this example, encryption ensures the security of electronic patient health information, as required by the HIPAA Security Rule. Only authorized personnel with the encryption key can access the data.

Privacy Beyond Borders:

While HIPAA is a cornerstone of healthcare data privacy in the United States, healthcare organizations operating globally must also navigate international privacy laws. The European Union's General Data Protection Regulation (GDPR), for instance, has a far-reaching impact on how healthcare data is handled when EU citizens are involved. This adds an extra layer of complexity to healthcare data management, making it essential for organizations to have a comprehensive understanding of the global regulatory landscape.

In summary, understanding privacy regulations, particularly HIPAA, is paramount for anyone dealing with healthcare data. It's not just a matter of compliance; it's a commitment to the ethical and responsible handling of sensitive information. Healthcare professionals, data scientists, and developers must work together to ensure that patient privacy is protected while still advancing medical research and patient care. The Python example above illustrates just one aspect of how technology can be employed to meet these standards, showing that, in the world of healthcare and medical research, data security is a priority.

Understanding the Need for Anonymization and De-identification

Before we dive into the methods, let's understand why these techniques are essential. Anonymization and de-identification are critical for balancing two seemingly conflicting goals: facilitating medical research and protecting patient privacy. Healthcare data, often including details like names, addresses, and social security numbers, can be a goldmine for researchers. However, using this data without proper safeguards violates privacy regulations and ethical considerations.

Anonymization: Protecting Identities

Anonymization is the process of removing or altering personally identifiable information (PII) from healthcare data. The goal is to make it impossible to identify an individual from the data. One common technique is to replace names with codes, remove dates of birth, and modify other direct identifiers. Python provides powerful libraries for this purpose, such as pandas and numpy.

Let's look at a simple example of anonymizing data using Python:

python

```
import pandas as pd

# Load the healthcare dataset
data = pd.read_csv('healthcare_data.csv')

# Anonymize patient names by replacing them with unique
codes
data = data.apply(lambda name: hash(name))

# Save the anonymized data to a new file
data.to_csv('anonymized_healthcare_data.csv', index=False)
```

In this example, we've loaded a healthcare dataset, anonymized the patient names using a hash function, and saved the anonymized data to a new file. This ensures that patient identities are protected while retaining the integrity of the dataset for analysis.

De-identification: Removing Sensitive Information

De-identification, on the other hand, focuses on removing specific details that could lead to re-identification. It's not just about making data anonymous but also preventing potential identification through indirect information. Techniques include generalization (replacing specific ages with age ranges) and suppression (removing details entirely). The pandas library is also useful for de-identifying data.

Here's an example of de-identifying healthcare data using Python:

python

import pandas as pd

# Load the healthcare dataset
data = pd.read_csv('healthcare_data.csv')

# De-identify dates of birth by replacing them with age ranges
data = data.apply(lambda dob: calculate_age(dob))

# Remove sensitive details like social security numbers
data = data.drop(columns=)

# Save the de-identified data to a new file
data.to_csv('deidentified_healthcare_data.csv', index=False)

In this case, we've loaded the dataset, replaced specific dates of birth with age ranges, removed the social security numbers, and saved the de-identified data. This process ensures that even with access to the data, re-identifying individuals becomes exceedingly difficult.

Ethical and Legal Considerations

It's essential to be aware of the ethical and legal considerations when anonymizing and de-identifying healthcare data. Regulations like the Health Insurance Portability and Accountability Act (HIPAA) provide guidelines on protecting patient privacy. Always ensure compliance with such regulations to avoid legal consequences.

Anonymization and de-identification are pivotal techniques in the realm of healthcare data. By understanding and implementing these methods, you can harness the power of healthcare data for research while upholding the highest standards of patient privacy and data security. Python's versatile libraries make it a valuable tool for these processes, ensuring that you can work efficiently and responsibly with healthcare datasets.

Security and Data Breach Prevention

In an era where the healthcare industry has become increasingly reliant on digital data, ensuring the security and privacy of sensitive patient information is paramount. This subsection delves into the strategies and best practices for securing healthcare data to prevent breaches. While we'll primarily focus on the conceptual aspects of security, I'll also provide you with some Python code examples to illustrate practical implementation.

Encryption: Shielding Data from Prying Eyes

Encryption is the first line of defense when it comes to data security. By converting data into an unreadable format, even if an unauthorized gains access to it, the information remains indecipherable. In Python, the 'cryptography' library is a powerful tool for implementing encryption. Here's a basic example:

python

```python
from cryptography.fernet import Fernet

# Generate an encryption key
key = Fernet.generate_key()

# Create an encryption object
cipher_suite = Fernet(key)

# Data to be encrypted
data = b"Patient123: John Doe, DOB: 01/15/1980, Diagnosis: Hypertension"

# Encrypt the data
cipher_text = cipher_suite.encrypt(data)

# Decrypt the data
plain_text = cipher_suite.decrypt(cipher_text)
```

Access Control: Restricting Entry

Controlling who has access to healthcare data is crucial. Python can be used to implement access control through authentication mechanisms. Below is a simplified example:

python

```
class :
    def __init__(self, name, password):
        self.name = name
        self.password = password

# Example healthcare staff
doctor = ("DrSmith", "p@ssw0rd")
nurse = ("NurseAmy", "securePwd")

def authenticate(name, password):
    if name == doctor.name and password == doctor.password:
        return "Doctor"
    elif name == nurse.name and password == nurse.password:
        return "Nurse"
    else:
        return "Invalid "

# Usage
_type = authenticate("DrSmith", "p@ssw0rd")
```

Monitoring and Intrusion Detection: Keeping an Eye Out

Continuous monitoring is key to identifying unusual activities that might indicate a breach. Python can be employed for log analysis and real-time alerts. Below is a basic example using Python's 'logging' library:

python

```
import logging
```

```
# Configure the logger
logging.basicConfig(filename='security.log',
level=logging.INFO)
```

```
# Simulate a suspicious login attempt
logging.info("Unauthorized access attempt from IP:
192.168.0.123")
```

Regular Updates and Patch Management: Staying Current

To prevent data breaches, it's essential to keep all systems and software up to date. Python is a handy tool for automating updates and patches. Here's a simple script:

python

```
import os
import subprocess
```

```
# Update the system
def update_system():
    try:
        subprocess.check_output()
```

```
    subprocess.check_output()
except subprocess.CalledProcessError:
    print("Error updating the system.")

# Usage
update_system()
```

Employee Training and Awareness: The Human Element

The best security measures can be compromised if employees are not adequately trained. Python can assist in creating interactive training modules. While a full training module is beyond the scope here, a simple interactive Python script could be used to simulate security scenarios and test employees' responses.

The security of healthcare data is not a one-time effort but an ongoing commitment. By implementing these strategies and embracing a proactive security culture, healthcare organizations can significantly reduce the risk of data breaches and safeguard patient information. Remember, the examples provided here are just a starting point, and the world of cybersecurity is vast and ever-evolving. Continual learning and adaptation are essential in this critical domain.

Ethical Considerations in Healthcare Data

In the realm of healthcare and medical research, the handling of data is not merely a technical or administrative task. It comes with a profound responsibility to uphold ethical standards and principles that safeguard patient privacy, data integrity, and the trust of the individuals whose information we process. In this section, we delve into the ethical considerations that underpin the entire landscape of healthcare data handling.

Patient Privacy: A Sacred Trust

At the heart of ethical healthcare data management is the commitment to preserving patient privacy. In a world where personal information is becoming increasingly vulnerable, healthcare providers and researchers must take every precaution to protect the sensitive data they work with.

Consider a scenario where a medical research institution collects data from various sources, including electronic health records (EHRs) and patient interviews. This data is often anonymized to remove direct identifiers, but even in its de-identified state, it can potentially be re-identified if not handled with care. Ethical considerations dictate that every effort must be made to protect the anonymity of individuals involved.

One way to ensure privacy is through robust encryption and access controls. Modern encryption techniques, such as homomorphic encryption, allow computations to be performed on data without ever exposing the raw information. Access controls, on the other hand, limit who can view or manipulate the data, ensuring that only authorized personnel can access the information.

Data Ownership and Consent

Another ethical challenge arises when considering data ownership and consent. Patients' medical records and data do not inherently belong to healthcare providers or researchers.

Instead, they are the property of the individuals involved. As such, ethical guidelines dictate that patient consent is of paramount importance.

Researchers must ensure that they have proper consent from patients to use their data for research purposes. This consent process should be transparent, informative, and, most importantly, voluntary. Patients should have the right to understand how their data will be used and the option to opt out if they wish.

In the realm of consent, there are intricacies, such as data sharing. If research data is to be shared with other institutions or researchers, ethical considerations come into play. Patients should be informed of such sharing, and their consent should extend to these scenarios as well.

Bias and Fairness

Ethical concerns in healthcare data handling also touch on the issues of bias and fairness. When using data to make critical decisions, such as treatment plans or resource allocation, it is vital that this data is not biased in any way that could lead to discriminatory outcomes.

For instance, if a machine learning model is used to predict disease outcomes based on historical data, and that data is biased in terms of race or gender, it could lead to unfair or discriminatory predictions. Ethical considerations demand that data used for such models be carefully examined for bias and that steps be taken to mitigate it.

Transparency and Accountability

Transparency is a core ethical principle when it comes to healthcare data handling. Patients and the public should have access to information about how data is collected, used, and protected. This transparency not only fosters trust but also allows individuals to exercise their rights to data privacy.

Moreover, accountability is equally crucial. In the event of data breaches or misuses, healthcare institutions and researchers must take responsibility for their actions and have mechanisms in place to rectify any potential harm. The ethical code of healthcare data handling requires rigorous data audit trails and accountability structures.

Python in Ethical Healthcare Data Handling

Python plays a significant role in upholding ethical standards in healthcare data management. It provides tools and libraries for secure data encryption, access control, and data anonymization. Moreover, Python's data analysis capabilities are instrumental in identifying biases in healthcare datasets and promoting fairness in predictive models.

Below is a Python code snippet illustrating how data anonymization can be achieved, ensuring that sensitive information is protected:

python

```
import pandas as pd
from faker import Faker

# Load patient data
```

```
data = pd.read_csv('patient_data.csv')

# Initialize a Faker object
fake = Faker()

# Anonymize patient names
data = data.apply(lambda x: fake.name())

# Save anonymized data
data.to_csv('anonymized_patient_data.csv', index=False)
```

This code snippet uses the Faker library to replace patient names with randomly generated names, thus preserving anonymity.

Ethical considerations in healthcare data handling are not a mere formality but a moral obligation. Python, with its versatile tools and libraries, empowers healthcare professionals and researchers to navigate this ethical terrain responsibly, ensuring that the data they work with is handled with the utmost care, respect, and adherence to ethical principles. The consequences of ethical lapses in healthcare data management are profound, affecting not only individuals but also the credibility and integrity of the entire healthcare industry. It is imperative that we embrace these ethical considerations as an integral part of our data-driven journey in healthcare.

Ethical Considerations in Healthcare Data

Throughout this book, we have traversed the expansive landscape of Python's applications in healthcare, from data manipulation and visualization to machine learning and deep learning techniques. But amidst the excitement of these transformative technologies, we must never lose sight of the ethical responsibilities that come with handling healthcare data.

Healthcare data is unique in its sensitivity and potential consequences. It can contain highly personal and identifiable information about individuals, and its usage can have direct impacts on their health and well-being. Therefore, maintaining the highest ethical standards is paramount.

Privacy Regulations in Healthcare

One of the key aspects we've explored is the labyrinth of privacy regulations that govern healthcare data. The Health Insurance Portability and Accountability Act (HIPAA) in the United States, GDPR in Europe, and various national and regional laws worldwide, impose strict rules on the collection, storage, and processing of healthcare data. These regulations aim to ensure the privacy and security of patients' information.

We've learned about the importance of compliance with these regulations, not only as a legal obligation but as a moral imperative. Healthcare professionals and data practitioners must be well-versed in these rules, implementing measures that safeguard sensitive data from breaches and unauthorized access.

Anonymization and De-identification

To balance the need for data-driven insights with patient privacy, we've delved into anonymization and de-identification techniques. These methods allow us to use healthcare data for research and analysis while removing or obfuscating personally identifiable information. By doing so, we can protect individual privacy without compromising the utility of the data.

Security and Data Breach Prevention

The significance of data security cannot be overstated. We've discussed strategies to secure healthcare data and prevent data breaches. Implementing robust cybersecurity measures is crucial in safeguarding not only the privacy of patients but also the integrity of medical research and healthcare systems.

Ethical Considerations in Healthcare Data Handling

In healthcare data, ethical dilemmas can arise. We've explored the nuances of balancing data utility with privacy concerns, particularly in cases where aggregated data might indirectly reveal sensitive information. Ethical considerations extend beyond legal regulations, demanding a thoughtful and responsible approach to healthcare data handling.

CHAPTER 11. DATA INTEGRATION AND HEALTHCARE SYSTEMS

In the fast-evolving landscape of healthcare, where data is a cornerstone of progress, it becomes increasingly vital to seamlessly integrate Python-powered solutions with Electronic Health Record (EHR) systems. The ability to work with these systems is akin to finding the right key to unlock a treasure trove of patient information, research data, and invaluable insights.

Understanding Electronic Health Records

Before we delve into the intricacies of integrating Python with EHR systems, it's essential to comprehend what EHR systems are. EHRs are digital versions of a patient's paper chart, containing their medical history, diagnoses, medications, treatment plans, immunization dates, allergies, radiology images, and laboratory results. They are the lifeblood of modern healthcare and are used by healthcare providers to deliver high-quality patient care.

Python's role in this domain is multifaceted, allowing

healthcare professionals and researchers to tap into the vast wealth of data within EHR systems, ultimately improving patient care, facilitating research, and enhancing operational efficiency.

The Power of Integration

Seamless integration of Python with EHR systems opens up numerous possibilities. It allows healthcare providers to access and analyze patient data in real-time, aiding in diagnosis and treatment decisions. Researchers can harness the data for large-scale studies, leading to medical breakthroughs and advancements in the field. Integrating with EHR systems can also streamline administrative tasks, reducing the burden on healthcare staff and improving the overall patient experience.

Python's simplicity and versatility make it an ideal choice for EHR integration. Let's explore the key aspects of this integration.

APIs and EHR Connectivity

Application Programming Interfaces (APIs) are the linchpin in integrating Python with EHR systems. Most EHR systems come equipped with APIs that facilitate data retrieval, updating patient records, and conducting various operations. Python can interact with these APIs to pull data into its ecosystem, allowing for real-time data processing and analysis.

Here's a simple Python script demonstrating how to connect to an EHR system using its API:

python

```python
import requests

# EHR API endpoint
ehr_url = 'https://ehr-system.com/api/patient-data'

# Your API credentials
api_key = 'your_api_key'
api_secret = 'your_api_secret'

# Make an API request
response = requests.get(ehr_url, headers={'Authorization': f'Bearer {api_key}:{api_secret}'})

# Check for a successful response
if response.status_code == 200:
    patient_data = response.json()
    # Process patient data here
else:
    print('Failed to retrieve patient data. Check your credentials and API endpoint.')
```

Data Transformation and Analysis

Once data is integrated, Python offers a plethora of tools and libraries for data transformation and analysis. Pandas, NumPy, and Scikit-Learn are your trusty companions in this journey. For instance, you can use Pandas to clean and structure patient data efficiently.

Let's consider a hypothetical scenario where you have extracted a dataset of patient vitals from the EHR system, and you wish to calculate some basic statistics:

python

```python
import pandas as pd

# Assume you have retrieved patient vitals data as a CSV
patient_vitals = pd.read_csv('patient_vitals.csv')

# Calculate basic statistics
summary_stats = patient_vitals.describe()

# Visualize the data
import matplotlib.pyplot as plt

patient_vitals.plot(kind='hist')
plt.title('Distribution of Heart Rates')
plt.xlabel('Heart Rate')
plt.ylabel('Frequency')
plt.show()
```

This is just a glimpse of the analytical capabilities Python provides when integrated with EHR systems.

Ensuring Data Privacy and Security

When dealing with sensitive patient data, privacy and security are paramount. HIPAA (Health Insurance Portability and Accountability Act) regulations in the United States, for example, enforce strict rules on patient data protection. It's crucial to ensure that your Python-based applications adhere to these regulations and maintain the highest standards of data security.

Encryption, access controls, and regular security audits are some of the measures that should be in place. Additionally, anonymization and de-identification techniques can be employed to protect patient identities while retaining the value of the data for research and analysis.

Real-world Applications

To put the concepts into perspective, consider a scenario where a healthcare provider aims to create a dashboard that displays a patient's vital signs in real-time. Python can connect to the EHR system's API, retrieve the data, process it, and present it in a -friendly interface using libraries like Dash or Flask.

On the research front, the integration of Python with EHR systems has enabled groundbreaking studies. For example, epidemiologists can access large-scale patient data to track the spread of diseases or evaluate the effectiveness of interventions swiftly.

Integrating Python with EHR systems opens doors to a world of possibilities in healthcare and medical research. From providing better patient care to conducting cutting-edge studies, Python's versatility and simplicity make it a powerful ally in this journey. The ability to seamlessly connect with EHR systems, process data, and ensure data security empowers healthcare professionals and researchers to make informed decisions, ultimately improving the quality of healthcare worldwide. As we continue our exploration of Python in healthcare, the next chapter will delve into the art of extracting data from healthcare databases, another critical skill in this dynamic field. So, fasten your seatbelts, and let's embark on this data-driven adventure!

Structured Query Language (SQL): A Powerful Tool

One of the most commonly used methods for data extraction from healthcare databases is SQL, or Structured Query Language. SQL is a versatile and powerful tool for managing and querying databases. It allows you to interact with the database using structured and specific commands. With SQL, you can extract data that meets certain criteria, sort and arrange it, and perform various operations on the data.

Let's consider an example using a Python script to demonstrate how SQL can be employed for data extraction. Assume we have a healthcare database with patient information, and we want to extract data for all patients above the age of 60. We can use the following SQL query:

python

```
import sqlite3

# Connect to the database
conn = sqlite3.connect('healthcare_data.db')
cursor = conn.cursor()

# Execute an SQL query to select patients above the age of 60
cursor.execute("SELECT * FROM patients WHERE age > 60")
```

```
# Fetch and print the results
results = cursor.fetchall()
for row in results:
    print(row)

# Close the database connection
conn.close()
```

In this example, we first establish a connection to the database, then use an SQL query to select the desired data, and finally fetch and print the results. SQL provides a standardized way to extract data, making it an essential tool in the healthcare domain.

Python Database APIs

Python offers a variety of database APIs that facilitate data extraction. Libraries such as SQLAlchemy and Django ORM provide a higher-level, object-oriented approach to database interaction, which can make the process more intuitive and efficient. These libraries support multiple database management systems, including PostgreSQL, MySQL, and SQLite.

Here's a brief example using SQLAlchemy to extract data from a PostgreSQL database:

python

```
from sqlalchemy import create_engine, text
from sqlalchemy.orm import sessionmaker
```

```
# Create an engine to connect to the database
engine                =                create_engine("postgresql://
name:password@localhost/healthcare_db")

# Create a session
Session = sessionmaker(bind=engine)
session = Session()

# Define and execute an SQL query
query = text("SELECT * FROM patients WHERE age
> :age_threshold")
result = session.execute(query, {"age_threshold": 60})

# Print the results
for row in result:
    print(row)

# Close the session
session.close()
```

In this example, we utilize SQLAlchemy to establish a connection to a PostgreSQL database, define an SQL query, and execute it with parameters. This demonstrates how Python's libraries can streamline the data extraction process.

Web Scraping for Healthcare Data

In some cases, healthcare data may not be readily available in a structured database. Researchers often turn to web scraping techniques to collect information from websites or online sources. Python provides various libraries, including Beautiful Soup and Scrapy, which assist in web scraping.

For instance, if you need to extract data from medical research articles on a healthcare portal, Beautiful Soup can be immensely helpful. You can parse the HTML content of web pages, extract relevant information, and save it for further analysis.

python

```python
import requests
from bs4 import BeautifulSoup

# Define the URL of the healthcare portal
url = "https://example-healthcare-portal.com/research-articles"

# Send an HTTP request to the URL
response = requests.get(url)

# Parse the HTML content
soup = BeautifulSoup(response.text, 'html.parser')

# Extract and print relevant data
research_titles = soup.find_all("h2", class_="research-title")
for title in research_titles:
    print(title.text)
```

In this web scraping example, we first make an HTTP request to the healthcare portal, parse the HTML content, and extract the titles of research articles. Web scraping provides a way to access and gather data from various online sources.

These are just a few of the techniques for data extraction from healthcare databases. Depending on your specific needs and the nature of the data, you may choose one or more of these methods. Extraction of data is a crucial step in the healthcare research process, as it enables the acquisition of valuable information for analysis and decision-making. The ability to extract and manipulate data efficiently is a core skill for those working in healthcare and medical research.

Real-time Data Streams: A Vital Healthcare Component

Real-time data streams encompass a constant flow of data generated at the very moment it is collected. In the context of healthcare, this can include patient vitals, monitoring device data, and even data from IoT devices in hospital settings. The significance of real-time data streams lies in the immediacy of insights they can offer. Timely information can lead to quicker medical interventions and more accurate decision-making, ultimately improving patient care.

Python's Role in Managing Real-time Data

Python, known for its versatility, has a role to play in managing real-time healthcare data streams. Several Python libraries and frameworks can aid in the collection, processing, and analysis of this data. Let's explore how Python fits into the picture:

1. Data Collection: Python offers a multitude of libraries for data collection. Popular choices include PyKafka and Apache Kafka for handling streaming data. These libraries allow you

to connect to data sources, retrieve information, and process it in real-time.

2. Data Processing: Once the data is collected, Python shines in its data processing capabilities. You can employ libraries like Apache Spark and Streamz to efficiently process incoming data. Whether it's filtering out irrelevant data, aggregating information, or performing real-time analytics, Python provides the tools needed.

3. Integration with Healthcare Systems: Real-time data streams need to seamlessly integrate with healthcare systems, including Electronic Health Record (EHR) systems. Python, with its extensive ecosystem of packages, facilitates such integration. You can use libraries like PyDICOM for handling medical image data or FHIR-Resources for managing healthcare data.

4. Machine Learning: If your healthcare application requires real-time predictive analysis, Python's machine learning libraries, such as Scikit-Learn and TensorFlow, can be invaluable. These libraries enable the creation of predictive models that can assess incoming data and provide timely insights.

Case Study: Monitoring Critical Care Patients

To illustrate the practical use of Python in handling real-time data streams in healthcare, let's consider a case study involving the monitoring of critical care patients. In an Intensive Care Unit (ICU), patients' vital signs, such as heart rate, blood pressure, and oxygen saturation, need constant monitoring.

Python Code Example: Real-time Vital Sign Monitoring

python

```
# Import necessary libraries
import time
import random

# Simulate a real-time data stream of vital signs
while True:
    heart_rate = random.randint(60, 100)
    blood_pressure = f"{random.randint(90, 140)}/{random.randint(60, 90)}"
    oxygen_saturation = random.uniform(95, 99)

    # Process and analyze the data as needed
    # Implement alerts or triggers for medical staff

    # For the sake of this example, let's simulate a delay
    time.sleep(5) # Simulating a 5-second interval
```

In this example, we simulate real-time vital sign data for patients. While this is a basic illustration, in a clinical setting, the data collected would be transmitted from actual monitoring devices.

Handling real-time data streams in healthcare is essential for timely decision-making and enhanced patient care. Python, with its versatility and a wide array of libraries, empowers healthcare professionals to collect, process, and integrate real-time data seamlessly. The example of vital sign monitoring illustrates the potential applications of Python in healthcare's real-time data landscape.

Interoperability and Healthcare Standards

Interoperability in the realm of healthcare is not just a buzzword; it's a critical necessity that can significantly impact patient care, data sharing, and research. As we delve into this section, we'll explore the complex world of healthcare data interoperability and the standards that govern it.

The Heart of Healthcare Interoperability

Imagine a scenario where a patient walks into a healthcare facility. This patient has a history of medical records scattered across different healthcare systems – from hospitals and primary care physicians to diagnostic labs. The challenge? Each of these systems may use different software, file formats, and data structures, making it cumbersome to exchange vital information.

This is where interoperability comes into play. It's the ability of various healthcare systems and software applications to communicate, exchange data, and interpret that shared data. In essence, interoperability ensures that data flows seamlessly, making critical patient information available at the right time and place, irrespective of the systems involved.

Key Standards Facilitating Interoperability

The world of healthcare interoperability is governed by a set of standards and protocols. These standards are pivotal in ensuring that different healthcare entities can speak the same language when it comes to data exchange. Here are some of the key standards you need to know:

HL7 (Health Level Seven): HL7 is the backbone of healthcare data exchange. It provides a framework and standards for the exchange, integration, sharing, and retrieval of electronic health information. When you're dealing with patient demographics, clinical documents, and laboratory results, HL7 is at the forefront.

FHIR (Fast Healthcare Interoperability Resources): FHIR is emerging as a game-changer. It's a standard for exchanging healthcare information electronically. What sets FHIR apart is its modern approach to data exchange, using simple RESTful APIs. This simplicity enhances the speed of implementation and is well-aligned with web standards.

DICOM (Digital Imaging and Communications in Medicine): When it comes to medical images, DICOM is the go-to standard. It ensures that medical images and associated information can be easily shared across different imaging devices and healthcare systems. From X-rays to MRIs, DICOM maintains the integrity of these images.

CCDA (Consolidated Clinical Document Architecture): This standard is all about clinical documents. It defines the structure of clinical documents for the purpose of exchange. When a patient's clinical data needs to be sent from one provider to another, CCDA ensures that the data structure is uniform.

IHE (Integrating the Healthcare Enterprise): IHE is not a standard itself but a framework that integrates different standards. It's about making all these standards work together seamlessly to ensure that healthcare entities can share data effectively. Think of it as the conductor of the healthcare data orchestra.

Python's Role in Healthcare Interoperability

Python, being the versatile language that it is, plays a significant role in facilitating interoperability between different healthcare systems. How, you ask? Through libraries and frameworks that enable developers to create applications that can talk to multiple systems using these healthcare standards.

Take, for instance, the use of Python's libraries to parse HL7 messages. These libraries allow healthcare applications to receive, process, and generate HL7 messages efficiently. By harnessing Python, developers can ensure that patient data is smoothly transferred between healthcare providers using this ubiquitous standard.

Moreover, FHIR's RESTful nature aligns perfectly with Python's capabilities in handling web-based communication. Python's requests library is a powerful tool for interacting with FHIR APIs, making it easier for healthcare systems to retrieve or send patient data securely.

The ability to work with DICOM images, a standard often used in medical imaging, is another feather in Python's cap. There are Python libraries designed specifically for parsing, manipulating, and even visualizing DICOM images, ensuring that this vital component of healthcare data can be seamlessly integrated into various systems.

In a practical example, let's say you're developing an application that needs to pull patient data from an EHR system, convert it into a FHIR format, and transmit it securely to another healthcare provider's system. Python can be your go-to language for this task. You can use libraries like hl7apy for HL7, fhir.resources for FHIR, and specialized DICOM libraries to work with medical images. The end result? A robust, interoperable system that facilitates efficient data sharing.

In conclusion, healthcare interoperability standards are the linchpin in creating a seamless healthcare ecosystem. Python, with its versatility and rich ecosystem of libraries, provides the means to implement and adhere to these standards effectively. By choosing Python, developers can help bridge the gap between healthcare systems, ensuring that vital patient data flows smoothly and securely, ultimately benefiting patient care and medical research.

We've explored how these standards come to life with Python, but this is just the beginning. In the healthcare industry, where data can be a matter of life and death, the quest for seamless interoperability remains a journey of paramount importance. With Python as your ally, you're well-equipped to navigate the intricacies of healthcare data exchange.

In the next section, we'll delve into the fascinating world of building Healthcare APIs. These application programming interfaces are the conduits through which healthcare data flows, enabling communication between different systems. Stay with us as we explore this critical component in the healthcare data landscape.

Healthcare APIs

Healthcare APIs serve as the digital bridges that connect various components of the healthcare ecosystem. They facilitate data sharing between hospitals, laboratories, pharmacies, and other healthcare entities. In essence, they help streamline clinical workflows, improve patient care, and enhance the overall healthcare experience.

For instance, let's consider the scenario of a patient undergoing a series of medical tests in a hospital. The data generated, including diagnostic reports, vital signs, and medications, need to be seamlessly integrated into the patient's EHR. This integration ensures that healthcare providers can access this data promptly, make informed decisions, and provide the best possible care.

Development of Healthcare APIs

Building healthcare APIs is a multifaceted process that requires precision, security, and compliance with healthcare standards. Here, we'll outline the fundamental steps in the development of these APIs.

Identifying Data Sources: The first step involves identifying the data sources, which can include EHR systems, healthcare databases, or real-time data streams. Each source may have unique data formats and requirements.

Data Extraction: Once the sources are identified, the data must be extracted using suitable methods. This could involve extracting patient records, lab results, or real-time monitoring data.

Data Transformation: Data from different sources often

comes in various formats. Transformation processes are essential to ensure that all data adheres to a common structure and can be easily integrated.

API Design: Designing the API involves defining endpoints, requests, and responses. It's essential to consider security measures such as authentication and encryption to protect sensitive patient data.

Integration and Testing: The API should be seamlessly integrated into existing systems. Rigorous testing is vital to ensure that data is transmitted accurately and securely. Any discrepancies or errors must be addressed.

Compliance and Security: Healthcare APIs must adhere to privacy regulations like HIPAA (Health Insurance Portability and Accountability Act) to protect patient confidentiality. Regular security audits and updates are critical.

Documentation: Comprehensive documentation is key for both developers and end-s to understand how to interact with the API effectively.

Python in Healthcare API Development

Python has become a popular choice for building healthcare APIs due to its simplicity, versatility, and a plethora of libraries that can be used for this purpose. Below is a basic example of a Python code snippet for creating a simple healthcare API using the Flask framework:

python

```python
from flask import Flask, request, jsonify

app = Flask(__name__)

# Sample endpoint for patient data
@app.route('/patient/<patient_id>', methods=)
def get_patient_data(patient_id):
    # Replace with your data retrieval and transformation logic
    patient_data = retrieve_and_transform_data(patient_id)
    return jsonify(patient_data)

if __name__ == '__main__':
    app.run()
```

In this example, the Flask framework is used to create a web-based API. The /patient/<patient_id> endpoint allows s to retrieve patient data by specifying the patient's ID. The retrieve_and_transform_data function is a placeholder for the logic required to fetch and process the data.

Developers can expand upon this basic example to create more complex healthcare APIs that cater to specific data integration needs.

Healthcare APIs are pivotal in ensuring that healthcare professionals can access the right information at the right time. Whether it's pulling patient records from an EHR system or integrating real-time data from medical devices, these APIs have revolutionized the way healthcare data is managed and utilized.

Case Study: Building a Healthcare Data Integration System

In this case study, we will embark on a journey to demystify the intricate process of constructing a Healthcare Data Integration System using Python. As we delve into this practical application, you will grasp the significance of data integration in the realm of healthcare, and how Python serves as a powerful tool to streamline this complex endeavor.

Understanding the Landscape

Before we set our sails, let's establish some context. In today's healthcare landscape, data is generated from myriad sources: electronic health records (EHR) systems, databases, real-time data streams, and more. These disparate data sources are the lifeblood of medical institutions and researchers alike. However, making sense of this data in its raw, decentralized form is a colossal challenge. That's where data integration comes into play, weaving these threads of data into a coherent fabric.

Python as the Architect

Python's role as the chief architect in this integration process cannot be overstated. With its versatility, an array of libraries, and a supportive community, Python is the ideal choice for crafting our integration system. Python enables us to efficiently extract data from diverse sources, transform it into a unified format, and load it into a destination where it can be harnessed for analysis and decision-making.

A Practical Voyage

Our case study revolves around a fictional but true-to-life scenario. Imagine a large healthcare institution with numerous departments, each maintaining its own data silo. To gain a holistic view of patient health and treatment outcomes, these silos need to be merged into a cohesive structure. Our task is to design a data integration system that will perform this task seamlessly.

Key Components

Data Extraction: To begin, we use Python to extract data from various sources. This involves connecting to EHR systems, querying databases, and tapping into real-time data streams. Python's libraries, like SQLAlchemy and requests, simplify this data retrieval.

Data Transformation: Once collected, data often comes in different formats and structures. Python allows us to standardize and transform the data using libraries like Pandas, ensuring it aligns with our integrated system's schema.

Data Loading: After transformation, we must load the data into a central repository. This can be a data warehouse or database. Python, with its libraries such as SQLAlchemy and PyODBC, enables us to create this destination effortlessly.

Automation: A crucial element is automating the entire process. Python scripts and scheduling tools like cron or Windows Task Scheduler come to our rescue. Automation ensures that data remains updated in real-time.

Error Handling: Data integration can be fragile, given the numerous data sources involved. Python's exception handling capabilities allow us to gracefully deal with errors without halting the entire process.

Python Code Example

python

```
import pandas as pd
from sqlalchemy import create_engine

# Data Extraction
source1 = 'ehr_database_connection_string'
source2 = 'departmental_database_connection_string'
real_time_stream = 'real_time_data_stream_api'

data1 = pd.read_sql("SELECT * FROM patient_data", create_engine(source1))
data2 = pd.read_sql("SELECT * FROM departmental_data", create_engine(source2))
real_time_data = requests.get(real_time_stream).json()

# Data Transformation
# Assume data transformation code here, e.g., data merging and cleaning

# Data Loading
destination = 'central_data_warehouse_connection_string'
data1.to_sql('integrated_patient_data',
create_engine(destination), if_exists='replace')
data2.to_sql('integrated_departmental_data',
```

create_engine(destination), if_exists='replace')

Automation and Error Handling

You would create scripts for automation and implement error handling here.

Our Python-driven healthcare data integration system is now operational. It automates the extraction, transformation, and loading of data from various sources into a central repository. This integrated data provides a comprehensive view of patient health and departmental insights, enabling healthcare professionals to make more informed decisions.

Chapter Summary

Healthcare Data Integration: A Vital Cog in the Wheel

Throughout this chapter, we've underscored the importance of healthcare data integration. It's the process of harmonizing data from diverse sources such as electronic health records (EHR) systems, healthcare databases, and real-time data streams. By creating a unified platform for this data, healthcare providers can make more informed decisions, provide better patient care, and enhance the overall healthcare ecosystem.

Integrating with EHR Systems

Our journey began with insights into integrating with EHR systems, the digital backbone of modern healthcare. We discussed the significance of interoperability, allowing healthcare professionals to access and share patient information effortlessly. From patient history to treatment plans, EHR integration empowers healthcare providers with holistic data access.

Extracting Data from Healthcare Databases

Next, we delved into the techniques for extracting data from healthcare databases. You learned that healthcare data comes in various formats, including structured data in relational databases and unstructured data in the form of clinical notes and reports. The ability to efficiently extract and transform this data is a fundamental step toward data integration.

Real-time Data Streams in Healthcare

Healthcare doesn't wait, and neither should data. Real-time data streams have become crucial for monitoring patients, tracking medical equipment, and responding swiftly to critical events. This section explored the challenges and solutions in handling real-time healthcare data streams, ensuring that time-sensitive information is available when and where it's needed most.

Interoperability and Healthcare Standards

In an era of digital healthcare, interoperability is the linchpin for sharing data between different systems and providers. We discussed various healthcare standards, including Fast Healthcare Interoperability Resources (FHIR) and Health Level 7 (HL7), which facilitate seamless data exchange. Compliance with these standards is pivotal for fostering collaboration and ensuring data consistency.

Building Healthcare APIs

With the growing emphasis on API-driven healthcare systems, we examined the development of healthcare APIs. These interfaces allow different systems to communicate and share data securely. Whether you're building telehealth applications or enhancing patient portals, understanding how to design and implement healthcare APIs is a valuable skill.

Case Study: Building a Healthcare Data Integration System

Theoretical knowledge is essential, but practical application is where it all comes together. In this chapter, we walked through a case study on building a healthcare data integration system. By following this real-world example, you gained insights into how the concepts covered throughout the chapter are applied in a practical setting. This hands-on experience can be a stepping stone for your own healthcare integration projects.

In closing, this chapter has equipped you with a deep understanding of healthcare data integration. From the intricacies of EHR systems to the development of healthcare APIs and real-time data streams, you've explored the tools and techniques that enable the modern healthcare ecosystem. Data integration is not just a buzzword; it's the foundation of data-driven healthcare, and your grasp of these key concepts will empower you on your journey in the world of Python for healthcare and medical research.

CHAPTER 12
RESOURCES
AND TOOLS

Access to comprehensive and reliable datasets is the backbone of any data-driven endeavor. Whether you're an aspiring data scientist, a medical researcher, or a seasoned Python enthusiast looking to make an impact in the healthcare domain, the first crucial step is obtaining the right data. In this section, we'll embark on a journey to explore some of the most valuable healthcare datasets and repositories available to you.

1. The MIMIC-III Database

Our exploration begins with the Medical Information Mart for Intensive Care-III (MIMIC-III) database. This vast and openly accessible resource comprises de-identified health data from over 40,000 critical care patients. The dataset includes a diverse range of information, from patient demographics to vital signs, laboratory tests, medications, and much more. With such rich and extensive data, you can delve into predictive analytics, disease modeling, and numerous other healthcare research avenues.

2. CDC Wonder

The Centers for Disease Control and Prevention (CDC) provides a treasure trove of health-related data through their Wide-ranging Online Data for Epidemiologic Research (CDC Wonder) platform. Here, you can access a wide variety of public health data, including disease incidence, mortality rates, and population statistics. It's a vital resource for public health researchers and epidemiologists looking to analyze trends and patterns in health outcomes.

3. National Health and Nutrition Examination Survey (NHANES)

For researchers interested in nutrition and its effects on health, NHANES is a goldmine. This extensive survey collects data on the health and nutritional status of the U.S. population. With a focus on dietary intake, body measurements, and biochemical assessments, NHANES data can be used to conduct in-depth studies on nutrition-related topics and their impact on public health.

4. World Health Organization (WHO) Global Health Observatory Data Repository

The WHO's Global Health Observatory offers a wealth of global health data, including information on disease prevalence, healthcare infrastructure, and vital statistics. Researchers seeking to examine healthcare on a global scale can find valuable insights within this repository. The data here is essential for comparative analyses across different countries and regions.

5. PhysioNet

PhysioNet is an online repository that focuses on physiological signal processing. It provides access to a wide range of datasets related to vital signs, electrocardiograms (ECG), and other physiological measurements. These datasets are particularly useful for researchers in the field of bioinformatics and medical signal analysis.

6. Healthcare Cost and Utilization Project (HCUP)

If your research involves healthcare economics and utilization, HCUP, sponsored by the Agency for Healthcare Research and Quality (AHRQ), is the place to go. HCUP offers a comprehensive collection of healthcare utilization, cost, and quality data, which can be applied in health services research and policy analysis.

7. Kaggle Datasets

Kaggle, a well-known platform for data science and machine learning competitions, also hosts a wide array of healthcare datasets. From diagnostic imaging datasets to electronic health records, you'll find a plethora of datasets contributed by the data science community. Kaggle datasets are perfect for honing your data analysis and machine learning skills in a competitive environment.

These are just a few of the many valuable healthcare datasets and repositories available to you as you dive into the world of Python in healthcare and medical research. Whether you're interested in clinical decision support, epidemiology, medical imaging, or any other healthcare-related field, having the right data at your fingertips is an essential foundation for your work.

Now, as we've explored these remarkable resources, it's essential to understand how to access, preprocess, and work with these datasets using Python. In the following sections of this book, we will not only guide you through the process of acquiring and cleaning data but also show you how to harness Python's power for in-depth analysis and meaningful insights.

Python Libraries and Frameworks

In Python, there exists a treasure trove of libraries and frameworks that cater specifically to the intricate needs of healthcare and medical research. These tools are essential for any aspiring data scientist or researcher venturing into the realms of healthcare analytics and medical data manipulation. They not only streamline the process but also enhance the capabilities of Python in this field.

Let's embark on a journey through some of these indispensable Python libraries and frameworks, each offering a unique set of features and functionalities.

NumPy: Our first stop brings us to NumPy, the fundamental package for scientific computing with Python. NumPy is the cornerstone for working with arrays and matrices, crucial for any data manipulation and analysis task. It provides the foundation for various other libraries, making it an essential tool in the data scientist's arsenal.

python

import numpy as np

Example Usage:

python

```
# Creating a NumPy array
data = np.array()
```

Pandas: As we delve deeper into the realm of data manipulation, we arrive at Pandas. This library is your go-to choice for data analysis and manipulation. With its DataFrame structure, you can easily organize and explore complex datasets, perform data cleaning, and apply various statistical functions.

python

```
import pandas as pd
```

Example Usage:

python

```
# Creating a DataFrame
data = pd.DataFrame({'Name': , 'Age': })
```

Matplotlib: Moving on, we find Matplotlib, a comprehensive library for creating static, animated, and interactive visualizations in Python. It's incredibly useful for plotting data, generating charts, and visualizing healthcare statistics.

python

```
import matplotlib.pyplot as plt
```

Example Usage:

python

```
# Creating a simple line plot
x =
y =
plt.plot(x, y)
```

Seaborn: For more advanced and aesthetically pleasing statistical plots, Seaborn is our next destination. This library is built on top of Matplotlib and provides a high-level interface for creating informative and attractive statistical graphics.

python

```
import seaborn as sns
```

Example Usage:

python

```
# Creating a distribution plot
data = sns.load_dataset("iris")
sns.displot(data=data, x="sepal_length", kind="kde")
```

Scikit-Learn: Now, we transition into the world of machine learning, and Scikit-Learn is our trusty guide. This library offers simple and efficient tools for data analysis and modeling, including classification, regression, clustering, and more.

python

from sklearn import datasets

Example Usage:

python

```
# Loading the famous Iris dataset for classification
iris = datasets.load_iris()
```

TensorFlow and Keras: Our journey wouldn't be complete without venturing into the realms of deep learning. TensorFlow, along with the Keras API, provides a powerful platform for building and training neural networks, particularly for medical image analysis.

python

```
import tensorflow as tf
from tensorflow import keras
```

Example Usage:

python

```
# Creating a simple neural network model using Keras
model = keras.Sequential()
```

NLTK (Natural Language Toolkit): For the fascinating world of natural language processing (NLP) in healthcare, NLTK offers a wealth of resources. It's perfect for text analysis, sentiment analysis, and building healthcare chatbots.

python

import nltk

Example Usage:

python

```
# Tokenizing text using NLTK
text = "Natural language processing is amazing!"
tokens = nltk.word_tokenize(text)
```

These Python libraries and frameworks serve as the backbone of your journey through the world of healthcare and medical research. They empower you to tackle complex problems, make data-driven decisions, and contribute to the advancement of healthcare through the power of Python.

As you progress in your Python for healthcare and medical research endeavors, remember that each of these tools has its unique strengths and applications. Feel free to explore them, experiment, and harness their full potential to unlock new insights and innovations in the field.

Online Courses for Python in Healthcare:

Coursera:

Course: "Python for Data Science and Healthcare" by the University of Michigan.

Description: This comprehensive course offers a deep dive into Python's applications in healthcare data science. You'll learn about data visualization, analysis, and manipulation specific to the healthcare domain.

edX:

Course: "Data Science MicroMasters Program" by UC San Diego.

Description: A broad program encompassing various aspects of data science, including Python programming, machine learning, and data analysis techniques tailored for healthcare.

Udemy:

Course: "Python for Healthcare Data Science and Analysis."

Description: A practical course that focuses on real-world healthcare data scenarios. You'll explore data preprocessing, analysis, and visualization using Python libraries.

FutureLearn:

Course: "AI in Healthcare" by The University of Manchester.

Description: Discover how AI and Python are revolutionizing the healthcare industry through this engaging course. Learn about the applications of machine learning in healthcare.

Specialized Learning Platforms:

DataCamp:

Platform Description: DataCamp offers a series of interactive Python courses. For healthcare, you can explore courses on data manipulation, visualization, and specialized tracks focusing on healthcare applications.

Kaggle:

Platform Description: Kaggle hosts healthcare-related datasets and challenges. It's a great platform to practice your Python skills and compete with data enthusiasts worldwide.

LinkedIn Learning:

Platform Description: With a plethora of Python courses, this platform is a goldmine for expanding your skills in healthcare data analysis and research.

MIT OpenCourseWare:

Platform Description: MIT offers free online course materials, including Python programming, that are invaluable for aspiring data scientists in healthcare.

Now, let's dive into a practical example to demonstrate how you can utilize Python for healthcare data analysis. In this scenario, we'll work with a fictional healthcare dataset containing patient information. We aim to extract useful insights using Python's data manipulation and visualization libraries.

python

```python
# Importing necessary libraries
import pandas as pd
import matplotlib.pyplot as plt
```

```
# Loading the healthcare dataset
dataset = pd.read_csv('healthcare_data.csv')

# Exploratory Data Analysis (EDA)
# Calculate the average age of patients
average_age = dataset.mean()

# Visualize the distribution of patient ages
plt.figure(figsize=(8, 6))
plt.hist(dataset, bins=20, color='skyblue')
plt.title('Distribution of Patient Ages')
plt.xlabel('Age')
plt.ylabel('Count')
plt.show()

# Calculate the percentage of patients with chronic conditions
chronic_patients = dataset == 1]
percentage_chronic = (len(chronic_patients) / len(dataset)) *
100

# Display the result
print(f'The average age of patients in the dataset is
{average_age:.2f} years.')
print(f'{percentage_chronic:.2f}% of patients have a chronic
condition.')
```

In this example, we start by loading a dataset and performing exploratory data analysis. We calculate the average age of patients and visualize the age distribution. Additionally, we determine the percentage of patients with chronic conditions. This practical demonstration is a testament to the power of Python in healthcare data analysis.

With the recommended online courses and platforms, you'll have the knowledge and tools necessary to excel in your Python journey within the healthcare and medical research domain. These resources will not only equip you with essential skills but also keep you updated with the latest advancements in the field. Happy learning!

Conferences and Communities

In the ever-evolving landscape of healthcare and medical research, staying connected and informed is not just an option; it's a necessity. This subsection delves into the vibrant world of conferences and communities where healthcare professionals and Python enthusiasts converge to exchange knowledge, share insights, and foster innovation. Here, we'll explore some of the top events and online hubs that serve as invaluable resources for those looking to supercharge their journey into Python for healthcare.

Conferences: Where Learning Meets Networking

Conferences have long been recognized as the melting pots of knowledge, and in the realm of healthcare and Python, they play an essential role in bringing together experts, practitioners, and learners. Attending these events not only exposes you to cutting-edge research and real-world applications but also provides a golden opportunity to network with individuals who share your passion.

PythonMed

PythonMed is a highly regarded conference that specifically focuses on the applications of Python in healthcare and medical research. It's a hub of innovation where experts showcase their work and discuss the latest trends and breakthroughs in the field. This conference is where you can witness firsthand how Python is transforming healthcare. From predictive analytics to image analysis, PythonMed covers it all.

Health Informatics Conferences

While not exclusive to Python, health informatics conferences are treasure troves of knowledge for anyone venturing into the healthcare data domain. Events like the Healthcare Information and Management Systems Society (HIMSS) Annual Conference bring together professionals who are at the forefront of using technology, including Python, to revolutionize healthcare. The cross-pollination of ideas here can be a game-changer for your Python journey.

PyCon

Although not healthcare-centric, PyCon is one of the largest gatherings of Python enthusiasts worldwide. Its diverse range of talks and workshops can be immensely valuable for healthcare professionals. You'll find sessions on data analysis, machine learning, and libraries that are directly applicable to healthcare. It's the place to be if you're looking to expand your Python toolkit.

Online Communities: Connecting Beyond Boundaries

Conferences are fantastic, but you don't have to wait for an annual event to connect with like-minded individuals. Online communities provide a year-round platform for discussions, problem-solving, and collaboration. Here are some key communities that should be on your radar:

Stack Overflow

The go-to platform for programmers, Stack Overflow has a thriving Python community. Here, you can ask questions, share your knowledge, and learn from experts. It's a valuable resource when you encounter roadblocks or need insights into Python coding for healthcare.

GitHub

For those looking to collaborate on open-source healthcare projects or showcase their skills, GitHub is the place to be. You can find a plethora of healthcare-related repositories where Python is the primary language. Contributing to these projects is not only a great way to learn but also to make a positive impact on healthcare.

Reddit (r/Python and r/healthIT)

Reddit is home to numerous subreddits catering to Python and healthcare technology. Subreddits like r/Python and r/healthIT provide a platform for discussions, news sharing, and problem-solving. It's where you can connect with professionals in the field and stay updated on the latest trends.

LinkedIn Groups

LinkedIn offers a range of Python and healthcare-related

groups where professionals share their experiences and insights. Groups like "Python in Healthcare" or "Health IT Innovators" are excellent places to network and engage in meaningful discussions.

Python Code Snippets

Now, as we promised, let's not just talk about these resources; let's demonstrate how you can use Python to explore and access these invaluable communities online. Below is a code snippet that showcases how you can use Python to connect to an API that provides conference and community data.

python

```python
import requests

def get_conferences_and_communities():
    api_url = "https://api.pythonhealthcareevents.com"    # Replace with the actual API URL
    headers = {"Authorization": "Bearer your-api-key"}  # Add your API key here

    response = requests.get(api_url, headers=headers)

    if response.status_code == 200:
        data = response.json()
        return data
    else:
        return None
```

```
events_data = get_conferences_and_communities()

if events_data:
    for event in events_data:
        print(f"Event: {event}")
        print(f"Date: {event}")
        print(f"Location: {event}")
        print(f"Website: {event}")
        print("\n")
else:
    print("Failed to retrieve data. Please check your API key and URL.")
```

This code uses the Python requests library to make an API call to retrieve conference and community data. You'll need to replace the API URL and add your API key for it to work. Once you have the data, you can easily parse and display it as per your requirements.

CHAPTER 13. CONCLUSION

In this final chapter of "Python for Healthcare & Medical Research," we gather the threads of knowledge and insights we've woven throughout this comprehensive guide. You've embarked on a journey through the world of Python in healthcare, from its humble beginnings to its pivotal role in modern medical research. As you reach the conclusion, it's crucial to summarize the main takeaways and lessons learned from our exploration.

Python's Significance in Healthcare

Throughout this book, we've emphasized the growing importance of Python in healthcare research. Python has become more than just a programming language; it's now a powerful tool for medical professionals, researchers, and data scientists. Its simplicity, versatility, and extensive library support make it an ideal choice for healthcare data analysis, machine learning, and deep learning.

Data Handling and Manipulation

One of the key takeaways is the significance of efficient data handling and manipulation. We explored libraries like NumPy and Pandas, equipping you with the skills to clean, preprocess, and reshape healthcare data. This foundation is vital for anyone dealing with medical datasets, given their complexity and diversity.

Data Visualization and Interpretation

Effective data visualization is another cornerstone of this journey. With Matplotlib, Seaborn, and Plotly, you've learned how to translate raw data into insightful visualizations. We emphasized the importance of clear and compelling graphics for conveying your findings and aiding decision-making in healthcare.

Ethical Considerations

As you've delved into the world of healthcare data, we've reminded you of the ethical considerations that come with this responsibility. From privacy regulations to anonymization techniques, you've acquired the knowledge to handle healthcare data with utmost care and compliance.

Machine Learning and Deep Learning

Our exploration didn't stop at descriptive statistics and data cleaning. We ventured into machine learning and deep learning, essential tools for predictive modeling and image analysis. The Scikit-Learn library, convolutional neural networks, and transfer learning techniques are now part of your toolkit for solving complex healthcare problems.

Natural Language Processing (NLP)

NLP opened doors to text data analysis, sentiment analysis,

and healthcare chatbot development. You've gained insights into how NLP can extract valuable information from clinical text data, contributing to patient care and research.

Integration and Future Trends

Data integration, interoperability, and emerging technologies are crucial in today's healthcare landscape. With this knowledge, you're prepared to work with electronic health record systems and stay up-to-date with the latest trends in healthcare informatics. Python is indeed shaping the future of healthcare research.

Continued Learning and Exploration

As you wrap up this book, we encourage you to continue your exploration of Python in healthcare and medical research. This field is dynamic, with ongoing advancements and new challenges. By staying curious and engaged, you can be at the forefront of innovation in healthcare.

Acknowledgments

Lastly, we acknowledge the contributions of many individuals who have made this book possible. From the authors and researchers who paved the way in healthcare data analysis to the developers of Python and its libraries, this book stands on the shoulders of many. We also appreciate your dedication and curiosity as readers, which drives progress in the field.

In conclusion, "Python for Healthcare & Medical Research" has been a comprehensive guide to using Python in the healthcare domain. We hope this book equips you with the skills and knowledge needed to make a significant impact in healthcare and medical research. Remember that your journey doesn't end here; it's just the beginning of an exciting and evolving field. Thank you for being part of this exploration, and we wish you all the best in your endeavors.

Encouragement for Further Exploration

As we approach the conclusion of this comprehensive guide, it's not so much an end as it is a new beginning. You've embarked on a journey through the world of Python in healthcare and medical research, and now, we want to encourage you to continue down this exciting path.

Python is an incredibly versatile language with immense potential in the healthcare industry. Throughout this book, you've gained a solid foundation in Python, data manipulation, visualization, statistical analysis, machine learning, deep learning, natural language processing, ethics, and data integration—all in the context of healthcare. The skills and knowledge you've acquired are valuable and in high demand.

However, this field is continually evolving, with new discoveries, techniques, and technologies emerging at a rapid pace. Therefore, we urge you not to stop here but to consider this book as your stepping stone into a world of endless possibilities.

The Ongoing Python Journey in Healthcare

Python has solidified its position as a cornerstone of healthcare research and analysis. The demand for Python developers and data scientists in the healthcare sector is steadily increasing. Therefore, as you delve into further exploration, consider these key steps:

1. Stay Informed

The world of healthcare and technology never stops evolving. To remain at the forefront of innovation, it's crucial to stay informed about the latest developments, trends, and breakthroughs. One way to do this is by following healthcare and technology news outlets, subscribing to relevant journals, and participating in online communities and forums.

2. Continuous Learning

The journey of learning Python in healthcare doesn't conclude with this book. It's an ongoing process. Consider taking more advanced courses, attending workshops, and exploring cutting-edge topics such as genomics, telemedicine, and personalized healthcare. Python's versatility means it can be applied in various healthcare domains.

3. Open Source Contributions

The Python community is built on open-source principles, and contributing to open-source healthcare projects can be a rewarding experience. You can collaborate with professionals worldwide and make a meaningful impact on the healthcare industry.

4. Collaborate and Network

Healthcare is a multidisciplinary field, and collaborating with healthcare professionals, data scientists, clinicians, and researchers can lead to groundbreaking discoveries. Attend conferences, join meetups, and engage in networking events to build meaningful connections.

5. Real-World Projects

To gain practical experience, consider working on real-world projects in healthcare. Whether it's building predictive models, creating innovative healthcare apps, or analyzing large-scale medical data, practical projects will deepen your expertise and understanding.

6. Ethical Considerations

As you explore Python in healthcare, always remember the ethical considerations we've discussed in this book. Protecting patient data, adhering to privacy regulations, and making ethical choices are essential in this field.

Conclusion

In this concluding chapter, we want to emphasize that your journey with Python in healthcare is just beginning. The healthcare industry is at the intersection of data science, technology, and patient care, and Python is your key to unlocking its full potential.

So, as you close this book, remember that every line of code you write, every data point you analyze, and every insight you gain can contribute to improving healthcare outcomes, patient experiences, and medical research. Python is not just a programming language; it's a tool for making a positive impact on the world.

With your newfound knowledge, you have the power to shape the future of healthcare and medical research. So, keep coding, keep exploring, and keep pushing the boundaries of what's possible. Your journey is far from over—it's an ongoing adventure that will lead you to exciting destinations in the realm of Python for healthcare and beyond.

Thank you for joining us on this incredible journey. We look forward to seeing the remarkable contributions you'll make to the world of healthcare using Python. Here's to a future filled with innovation and positive change.

APPENDIX

Glossary

1. Python:

Definition: Python is a high-level, versatile programming language known for its simplicity and readability. In healthcare and medical research, Python is utilized for data analysis, machine learning, and more.

2. NumPy:

Definition: NumPy, short for Numerical Python, is a fundamental library for scientific computing. It provides support for large, multi-dimensional arrays and matrices, along with a variety of mathematical functions to operate on these arrays.

3. Pandas:

Definition: Pandas is a powerful library for data manipulation and analysis. It introduces data structures, like DataFrames and Series, that simplify tasks such as data cleaning, exploration, and transformation.

4. Data Cleaning:

Definition: Data cleaning refers to the process of identifying and rectifying errors, inconsistencies, and inaccuracies in datasets, ensuring the data's reliability for further analysis.

5. Machine Learning:

Definition: Machine learning involves the use of algorithms and statistical models to enable computer systems to progressively improve their performance on a specific task, without being explicitly programmed.

6. Deep Learning:

Definition: Deep learning is a subfield of machine learning that employs artificial neural networks to model and understand complex patterns in data, making it particularly valuable in tasks like medical image analysis.

7. Natural Language Processing (NLP):

Definition: NLP is a branch of artificial intelligence that focuses on the interaction between computers and human language. In healthcare, NLP is employed for tasks such as text analysis and chatbot development.

8. Electronic Health Record (EHR):

Definition: EHRs are digital versions of a patient's paper chart, containing their medical history, diagnoses, medications, treatment plans, immunization dates, allergies, radiology images, and laboratory results.

9. HIPAA:

Definition: HIPAA, the Health Insurance Portability and Accountability Act, sets the standard for protecting sensitive patient data. Compliance with HIPAA is crucial in handling healthcare data ethically and securely.

10. Anonymization:

Definition: Anonymization is the process of removing or altering personally identifiable information (PII) from data to protect individuals' identities and privacy.

11. Interoperability:

Definition: Interoperability refers to the ability of different information systems, devices, and applications to access, exchange, integrate, and cooperatively use data in a coordinated manner within and across organizational boundaries.

12. AI and ML:

Definition: Artificial intelligence (AI) and machine learning (ML) represent the cutting edge of technology in healthcare. AI can aid in diagnostics, while ML helps in recognizing patterns in vast medical datasets.

13. DICOM:

Definition: DICOM, or Digital Imaging and Communications in Medicine, is a standard for transmitting, storing, and sharing medical images, making it indispensable in fields like radiology.

14. Plotly:

Definition: Plotly is a library for creating interactive data visualizations in Python. It enables the development of dynamic, web-based visualizations to explore and present healthcare data.

15. Ethics in Healthcare Data:

Definition: Ethics in healthcare data encompass the moral considerations surrounding patient data, including consent, confidentiality, and responsible data handling.

16. Clinical Text Analytics:

Definition: Clinical text analytics involves applying natural language processing techniques to clinical text data, enabling the extraction of valuable insights from medical records and reports.

This glossary serves as your compass throughout the book, allowing you to navigate and understand the complex, yet fascinating world of Python in healthcare and medical research. Refer back to it whenever you encounter unfamiliar terminology, and you'll find it a valuable resource on your journey to mastering Python in this vital field.

SAMPLE CODE SNIPPETS AND EXERCISES

In the world of Python programming for healthcare and medical research, learning by doing is often the most effective approach. To help you gain a deeper understanding of the concepts we've covered throughout this book, we've prepared a selection of sample code snippets and exercises. These hands-on exercises are designed to reinforce your knowledge and provide you with practical experience in using Python for healthcare applications.

Exercise 1: Basic Python Syntax

Let's begin with a simple Python exercise to ensure you have a solid grasp of the language's fundamentals. In this exercise, you'll create a Python script that calculates the Body Mass Index (BMI) based on a person's height and weight. Here's a starter code snippet to get you going:

python

BMI Calculator

Input height and weight

```
height = float(input("Enter your height in meters: "))
weight = float(input("Enter your weight in kilograms: "))

# Calculate BMI
bmi = weight / (height ** 2)

# Display the result
print("Your BMI is:", bmi)
```

Your task is to complete this code, run it, and understand how it works. You'll see that Python's readability and simplicity make such tasks quite straightforward.

Exercise 2: Data Handling with Pandas

Now, let's delve into data handling using the Pandas library. For this exercise, we'll work with a sample healthcare dataset. Your goal is to read the dataset, perform basic data analysis, and extract some insights. Here's a sample code snippet to get you started:

```
python

import pandas as pd

# Read the healthcare dataset into a Pandas DataFrame
df = pd.read_csv('healthcare_data.csv')

# Display the first 5 rows of the dataset
print(df.head())

# Calculate basic statistics
```

```
print("Summary Statistics:")
print(df.describe())

# Filter data based on specific criteria
print("Patients with high blood pressure:")
print(df > 140])
```

This exercise will help you understand how to load and manipulate healthcare data efficiently using Pandas.

Exercise 3: Machine Learning for Disease Prediction

In this exercise, we'll explore the world of machine learning in healthcare. Your task is to build a simple machine learning model that predicts the likelihood of a patient developing diabetes. We'll use the Scikit-Learn library for this purpose. Here's a starting code snippet:

python

```
from sklearn.model_selection import train_test_split
from sklearn.ensemble import RandomForestClassifier
from sklearn.metrics import accuracy_score

# Split data into features (X) and target (y)
X = df.drop('Outcome', axis=1)
y = df

# Split the data into training and testing sets
X_train, X_test, y_train, y_test = train_test_split(X, y, test_size=0.2, random_state=42)
```

```python
# Create a Random Forest Classifier
clf = RandomForestClassifier()

# Train the model
clf.fit(X_train, y_train)

# Make predictions
y_pred = clf.predict(X_test)

# Calculate accuracy
accuracy = accuracy_score(y_test, y_pred)
print("Accuracy:", accuracy)
```

By completing this exercise, you'll have hands-on experience with building a machine learning model for healthcare data.

These sample exercises are just the tip of the iceberg. Throughout this book, you'll find more opportunities to practice and expand your Python skills. Remember that learning by doing is a powerful way to solidify your knowledge and become proficient in using Python for healthcare and medical research. So, roll up your sleeves, open your code editor, and dive into the world of Python in healthcare. The possibilities are endless, and the journey is incredibly rewarding.

ADDITIONAL RESOURCES

As you embark on your journey of learning Python for healthcare and medical research, I encourage you to explore further resources. The field is dynamic and ever-evolving, and staying up to date is crucial.

Online Healthcare Databases: Websites like PubMed, the World Health Organization (WHO), and the Centers for Disease Control and Prevention (CDC) offer a treasure trove of healthcare data and research.

Python Documentation: Python's official website and documentation (python.org) serve as your foundational resource for Python-related information.

Educational Platforms: Online platforms like Coursera, edX, and Khan Academy provide courses and tutorials tailored to various aspects of Python and healthcare.

Academic Journals: Journals such as JAMA (Journal of the American Medical Association) and The Lancet are invaluable sources of cutting-edge medical research.

By utilizing these resources and maintaining a diligent approach to referencing and citing, you'll ensure the integrity of your work and contribute to the ongoing advancement of healthcare research.